GROWING UP:
PASTORAL NURTURE
FOR THE LATER YEARS
Thomas B. Robb, ThD

AN ADVANCE REVIEW

"Must reading for those who work with or care about older adults. It takes into account the findings of developmental research but moves the reader a step beyond to the more personal, spiritual dimensions of growing up and growing old. Church professionals in the field of aging will find it helpful in shaping religious programs for aging persons."

Roy H. Ryan, DMin
Educational Consultant and Older Adult Ministry Specialist
Nashville, Tennessee
Former Director of Education and Ministry with Older Adults
General Board of Discipleship
The United Methodist Church, Nashville, Tennessee

HAWORTH Religion, Ministry & Pastoral Care
William M. Clements, PhD
Senior Editor

New, Recent, and Forthcoming Titles:

Growing Up: Pastoral Nurture for the Later Years by Thomas B. Robb

Religion and the Family: When God Helps edited by Laurel Arthur Burton

Keeping Mind and Body Together by Wm. Michael Clemmer

Growing Up
Pastoral Nurture
for the Later Years

Thomas B. Robb, ThD

The Haworth Press
New York • London • Sydney

1991

The Haworth Press, Inc., 10 Alice Street, Binghamton, NY 13904-1580
EUROSPAN/Haworth, 3 Henrietta Street, London WC2E 8LU England
ASTAM/Haworth, 162-168 Parramatta Road, Stanmore (Sydney), N.S.W. 2048 Australia

Library of Congress Cataloging-in-Publication Data

Robb, Thomas B.
  Growing up: pastoral nurture for the later years / Thomas B. Robb.
    p.   cm.
  Includes bibliographical references and index.
  ISBN 1-56024-072-5 (alk. paper). — ISBN 1-56024-073-3 (pbk. : alk. paper)
    1. Church work with the aged. 2. Aged—Religious life. 3. Christian life—1960- I. Title.
BV4435.R62   1991   91-7735
259'.3—dc20   CIP

CONTENTS

ABOUT THE AUTHOR

Thomas B. Robb, ThD, is currently Pastor of the Culver City Presbyterian Church in Culver City, California. In 1988, he became the Executive Director of the National Interfaith Coalition on Aging, through which 25 denominational agencies — Protestant, Catholic, Orthodox, and Jewish — work cooperatively. While serving as Director of the Office on Aging, Presbyterian Church (USA), from 1981-1989, Dr. Robb developed program resources and trained leaders for ministries with older adults. He has also served as Program Director in aging policy studies and training at the National Council on Aging, Assistant Professor of Pastoral Ministry at the Iliff School of Theology, and Director of Advanced Pastoral Studies at the San Francisco Theological Seminary. Dr. Robb is the author of *Senior Center Administration* (Washington: National Council on the Aging, 1978), *Senior Center Operation* (Washington: National Council on the Aging, 1978), and *The Bonus Years: Foundations for Ministry with Older Persons* (Valley Forge: Judson Press, 1968).

Preface

My fellow church members often seem to regard their own and others' aging as something shameful, a change for the worse that wasn't supposed to happen. They seem to regard every wrinkle or gray hair as a badge of dishonor. In this kind of thinking, they differ not a whit from other Americans for whom signs of the advancing years are tantamount to a lack of patriotism; for this is the land of the free (read *young*) and home of the brave (read *attractive*).

Congregations, and their pastors, devote disproportionate energies and resources to reviving or propping up church schools and youth programs. They seem unaware that these institutions are shrinking not so much for want of good leadership or creative programming as simply for want of enough young people to swell their ranks to former proportions. For nearly a quarter century, Americans, especially those of middle and upper income strata, have not been producing enough children to replace themselves.

When congregations reorganize their ministries in response to the growing numbers of older adults in their pews, the results seem to differ little from the offerings of the senior center down the street. There are classes, luncheons and trips to while away the leisure hours, phone calls, home delivered meals and blood pressure checks to offset the difficulties that attend growing older. Seldom are the faithful challenged to wrestle with the implications of the older believer's vocation in the context of empty nest or retirement.

Over the twenty-two years since I wrote *The Bonus Years*, I have been privileged to teach seminarians about pastoral ministry with older adults, train the management staff for a new church retirement home, write training manuals for senior center and nutrition site managers, develop program resources and train a network of consultants for my denomination's ministries with older adults. I have worked in thirty project sites with older adult leaders and pastors, developing and testing new approaches to older adult ministry.

The conclusions that have emerged in my own thinking over these years form the foundation upon which this book is based:

1. *Old age is supposed to happen.* Theoretical models that posit such processes as entropy, a genetic clock, or simple wear and tear, as the explanation for human aging will no doubt help us to understand how aging occurs, but offer no final explanation as to why it happens. Even a casual reading of scripture, especially the Old Testament, points to the reality that old age is part of the divine plan for human life.

Aging is part of creation's normal processes; all living species age. Contemporary medical science has not lengthened the span of years humans may live, only brought under control some of the things that, in the past, have unduly shortened life. Advances in sanitation, nutrition, the prevention of infectious disease, and improved care of those suffering from heart disease, cancer and diabetes, have only made it possible for more of us to survive childhood and live to an advanced age.

2. *The future belongs to the old.* Longevity has steadily increased in this century, from an average of 47 years in 1900, to an average of 77 years in 1989, and will continue to increase well into the next century. Further medical advances, and the continued aging of the *baby boom* generation, could possibly result in an average life span of 90 years by 2025.

The availability of inexpensive and reasonably safe birth control, combined with affluent industrial society's preference for small families and spreading concern about earth's capacity to sustain life for a continually expanding population, have lowered fertility rates almost everywhere. In most industrial societies, fertility has remained significantly below the replacement level for a quarter century. Some nations have set a limit on the number of children a family may have. Never again will any population be likely to be made up of such a large proportion of young children and adolescents as we have known in the past.

3. *Our vocation as people of faith is lifelong.* During childhood and adolescence we are taught the lore of our faith and the disciplines by which it is lived. In young adulthood we are distracted by

the demands of growing families and expanding careers, or simply by the necessity of supporting ourselves. Only as we lay aside the roles of parent and worker can we devote mature experience and energy to any of life's pursuits. Painters, writers, scholars, and poets often produce their best work late in life. Michelangelo, Casalls, Picasso, and Sarton are prime examples. What delights Gershwin, Shelley, and Keats might have left us had they lived into their seventies. Those acts for which Abraham, Sarah, Moses, John XXIII, and Mother Theresa are remembered and beloved all occurred late in life. It is more often in the later years that maturity of skill, knowledge and judgment are equal to the demands of the faith. Old age may therefore be that time when each of us is called and enabled, as never before, to respond to God's leading with creativity and insight.

The advancing years bring more than maturity of skill and knowledge. The limitations of our bodies and the exigencies of life in an imperfect environment often bring illness, diminished strength, and loss of function, thus lessening our capacity for discipleship. Yet our call is lifelong, and the limitations imposed by such misfortune do not exempt us from its urgency.

The congregation and its spiritual leaders thus face a dual challenge. They must employ as much, or perhaps more, diligence and skill fitting us for discipleship in our later life than they did when we were young. They must also enable us to cope with and overcome those facets of life that limit the fullest expression of our discipleship.

The experience of those older adults who took part in the Presbyterian Church's *Gift of a Lifetime Project* underlines the importance of discipleship in our later years. As they began their work of developing new ministries in congregations, often far from home, almost every one of the forty volunteers said, "This is the first time since I retired that my church has asked me to do something important." As they completed their two year projects, many said, "This has been the most demanding work I've undertaken in a long time, and the most important."

The *Gift of a Lifetime Project* volunteers, with whom I have shared portions of this book during their training seminars, have helped refine my understanding of later life. More importantly, by their example, they have reinforced my belief in the significance I believe God intends for our old age. For us as believers, there must be more to life than kids and careers, more to old age than shuffleboard and bingo. This book is about the tasks of pastor and congregation in making that happen.

NOTE

Quotations from Scripture are, unless otherwise noted, from the *Today's English Version (Good News Bible)*, Copyright by American Bible Society, 1966, 1971, 1976.

Chapter 1

Growing Up

> When I was a child, my speech, feelings, and thinking were all those of a child; now that I am a man, I have no more use for childish ways.
>
> — I Corinthians 13:11

One day, when I was very small, Uncle Paul asked me, "What do you want to be when you grow up?" Over the next few years, that question was to be repeated many times in conversations with grandparents, aunts and uncles. Each time I tried to answer it, I gained some understanding of what being grown up might mean. In time, I developed an agenda for growing up. It was based on a series of assumptions that would remain with me for more than fifty years: (a) that I was not yet grown up, but someday would be; (b) that when I grew up I would get to do what I wanted; and (c) that what grownups do is raise children and go to work.

Someday I will be grown up. After three or four such discussions, I began to realize that I was moving inexorably toward a time known as *grown up*. At first, I wasn't sure just when or how *grown up* began. I learned that dressing myself and tying my own shoes were marks of being *grown up*. One day Mother told me that when I was six I would be *grown up enough* to cross the street by myself and go to school. Sometime later, I learned from one of the older children that when I turned twelve, I would have to pay *grown up* prices on the elevated, and to see the latest episode of "Flash Gordon" at our neighborhood theater on Saturdays.

When I learned to dress myself and tie my shoes, when I went to school, and even later when I became twelve, I discovered that I wasn't *grown up* yet. I looked forward then to becoming sixteen, when I could get a drivers' license and my own jalopy. I was sure I

1

would then be *grown up enough* to decide where I wanted to go, when and with whom.

When I finally did reach sixteen, I couldn't afford a car of my own, and Father said I wasn't *grown up enough* to be entrusted with his. I then looked forward to being seventeen, when I could marry or join the Navy without my parents' permission, and then to eighteen, when I could legally buy and smoke cigarettes. I didn't marry or join the Navy that year, but I did take up smoking a pipe. Even so, I still wasn't *grown up*. At that point I decided that at twentyone, when I could vote and buy liquor, I would surely be *grown up*.

When I am grown up I can do what I want to do. Being able to decide for myself whether to get up, put on clean socks, study my geography, or go to school, was a future I had longed for since I was small. In the interim, I had to put up with parents, teachers, and a truant officer whom I never saw. They had definite ideas about what I should do with my time. Moreover, they had both power and authority sufficient to make me comply with their wishes. So I made peace with my circumstances and bided my time.

As I reached each of the ages at which I expected to be *grown up*, I was confronted with a dilemma. I could be *grown up* enough to dress myself and tie my own shoes yet not enough to do all that I wanted. I would pay the same prices as adults, yet not share their freedom of deciding where to go or which movie to see.

Even when I became twenty-one, I did not attain the freedom to do what I wanted. I graduated from college and moved out of my parents' house. I also married and began my studies for the ministry. In the place of parents, I now had a wife, a mother-in-law and a new set of teachers to deal with. There was also a presbytery committee weighing my candidacy for the ministry. I also had a draft board to think about because of U.S. involvement in Korea. They all had ideas about how I should make use of my time, and held considerable influence and authority over my life.

Soon I had children. As they grew, I found they too had expectations of how I would spend my time, and a certain amount of influence (especially when they joined forces with their mother or their grandparents). As adults with their own households and families, they still voice their expectations about how I should make use of vacations and holidays, and whether I see my grandchildren often enough.

While the children were still young, I finished seminary, passed my examinations, was ordained and installed as a pastor. Employed fulltime at the profession of my choosing, I found I still had to deal with the expectations, power and authority of others. In my case, it was the members and officers of the congregations I served, and the presbytery under whose authority I labored. Had I chosen a different line of work, I would have been accountable to customers or clients, a supervisor or manager, a board of directors or stockholders. Eventually, I too would deal with many of these.

When I am grown up, I will be a parent and a worker. From those early conversations of my childhood, I always assumed that I would one day be a parent. If I had to guess what my first answer was—about what I would be when I grew up—it was probably: "I'm going to be a daddy."

The little I knew about what grownups do was learned by observing my parents and my grandparents. I watched my mother and my grandmother cook and clean house, and went along when they shopped for food or clothes. Most days my father and my grandfather dressed in suits and left the house after breakfast, returning just before dinner. Sometimes Father stayed home and fixed things or sat at the dining table with a lot of papers spread before him. Sometimes I wore my good clothes and he took Mother and me to church. When I was still very young, I understood that someday I would do what my father did. How I knew that I would not cook and clean house and go shopping, as my Mother did, I am not sure but I knew.

In time, my answers reflected a growing awareness that I would eventually take up some sort of career. While I was still quite small I learned that when my father wore a suit and was away all day, he went *to work*. I didn't know what kind of work he did—even as an adult I understood little about what he did as a banker. I also remember visiting my grandfather's office. I watched him write with a long yellow pencil, talk on the telephone, and speak to a young woman who made strange marks on her notebook while he talked. By watching them, I understood that when I grew up I too would go to work.

My earliest notions of choice occupations probably reflected the romance children associate with certain kinds of work. Most likely, I spoke at first of becoming a policeman, fireman, mailman, an ice or milk wagon driver, or a conductor on the elevated trains which I loved to ride. A girl of my generation would probably have spoken of becoming a nurse or a teacher, or perhaps a secretary.

As a teenager, when others were talking of becoming doctors, lawyers, mechanics, plumbers, I narrowed my choices to electronic engineer (which my best friend planned to become) or parish pastor, which I had encountered when my parents became involved in starting a new church. Throughout high school, I waffled between these two careers — about which I knew little and understood less — and finally chose the latter.

Having thus become twenty-one, married, had children and begun my life's work, I assumed I was, at last, *grown up*. I was not prepared for what was to follow!

MY AGENDA HAS CHANGED

When I was forty-nine, the last of my five children assumed responsibility for her own support and established her own household. I had, at that point, completed one of the two major tasks on my agenda for growing up. By this time, the older children had married and there were several grandchildren. Nonetheless, I was, for all practical purposes, finished with the day-to-day, hands-on business of raising children. I was done with tying shoelaces, combing hair, packing lunches, dispensing allowance, and all the other tasks which occupied my time over more than a quarter century.

My concern for my children had not changed, only my day-to-day relationship with them. Any one of them might, out of personal need, return to my household for a time. It would be as an adult, however, not as a child. I might offer guidance from my longer experience, but not the kind of nurture I had once provided. I might resume some degree of oversight during a time of need, but not the complete responsibility that had once been mine. I had done with raising children. The passing years had turned them all into adults.

Now, at fifty-eight, I am within a few years of completing the other principal task in my agenda for *growing up*. Thanks to Social Security and my church pension plan, I anticipate retiring with full benefits in a few more years. These days, Americans retire at an average age of sixty-two. I will be eligible for reduced retirement benefits at age sixty-two, just four years hence. If I worked for a large corporation, I might be offered an early retirement option any day now.

I look forward to retiring. I may rock a little, but not for long. I expect to be busy, like many of the retired people I know. Nonetheless, I will no longer be obliged to work to support myself and my family. Even if I want to continue to work, I may find it difficult to do so. Employers are likely to devalue the skills I have acquired over forty years, in preference for the less costly experience of a younger worker who can stay with them longer than I might.

When I have finished with raising children, and have retired, I should, at last, be *grown up*. According to the agenda I worked out in my childhood, I will finally get to do what *I* want. That agenda does not, however, spell out what it is that I want to do with my life next.

Conventional wisdom divides life into three discrete stages: education, work, and leisure. Education is considered preparation for work, and leisure its reward. Work is considered the proper occupation for adult males, and unmarried females. Small amounts of learning and leisure can be accommodated within this period, on the premise that they contribute to effective work. Longer periods of either learning or leisure tend to be viewed as abdication or shirking of adult responsibility.

As I approach retirement, I find that I lack enthusiasm for a period of twenty years devoted solely to leisure. I value the rich variety of leisure activities that await me. I yearn for the time to *do what I want* without answering to any authority with its own agenda for my days. I am not, however, prepared to spend all my time at play.

It is the rhythm of education, work and leisure that has made my adult years both productive and exciting. I have learned to value education for its own disciplines and as an end in itself. I am not prepared to give it up because my years as a worker are drawing to a close. I have learned to value work also for its own methods, and as a worthwhile activity in itself, apart from its utility in keeping a roof over my head and bread on my table. I am not prepared to give it up even though the income from social security and my pension may be adequate for my needs.

The agenda for my adult years which I adopted in my youth is now demonstrably inadequate. How can I continue to be creative and productive if I stop learning and working? Of what worth is my life if I am neither creative nor productive? Clearly, I misunderstood the nature of adult life. Being *grown up* is not a state or status we will one day achieve. *Growing up* is a lifelong process we never finish. It must continue to the very threshold of the grave — and beyond.

Biologists now think humans could live 120 years if there were no wars, disease, accidents or pollution. That seems to be what God had in mind, too. "I will not allow people to live forever; they are mortal. From now on they will live no longer than 120 years" (Genesis 6:3). Very few actually live 120 years, but at fifty-eight, I can reasonably expect to live another twenty-five or thirty years. This last third of my life isn't part of that agenda I developed when I was young.

Parenting and work are essential adult tasks, but they don't require 120 years. Unless most of us bear and raise children, the human species will soon die out. Even if our children go to college, and on to graduate study, before they assume responsibility for themselves, we can finish raising the next generation by the time we are forty-five to fifty-five years old. Unless many of us work, there will be no food to eat, water to drink, clothes to wear, nor houses to live in. Our society has decided, nonetheless, that it is enough for us to work until we are fifty-five to sixty-five years old.

Parent and worker are adult roles deeply rooted in western culture. The expectation of living fifteen or twenty years after I have completed both primary adult roles forces me to ask myself whether or not they are all that being an adult is about. If I have the capacity to live 120 years, and a reasonable expectation of living eighty or ninety, am I to be content with finishing the essential business of life by the time I am sixty or sixty-five?

Parenting, after all, affords little opportunity for uniqueness and creativity. Each child is genetically and environmentally unique, yet family life is remarkably the same from one household to the next. There are not more than a dozen or so standard plots for American family life. That's why television situation comedies and comic strips about family life are funny. Their experiences are like our own or our neighbor's. Sometimes it seems as though the writers have been looking in our windows or listening at our keyholes.

Jobs, too, are more alike than different, and so are the organizations we work for. Work involves mostly reading, writing, listening, talking, counting, figuring, labeling, classifying, giving and following instructions, and similar basic tasks. All the thousands of job titles only reflect slightly different combinations of such tasks. In our work, we must all deal with or be accountable to owners, managers, subordinates, customers, and the like, whatever else we may call them.

If biologists and Genesis 6:3 are both correct, then God has made us to live much longer than necessary to replace ourselves and do whatever work is needed for survival. Medical skill and modern technology have not *lengthened* life in recent years, only brought under control or eliminated some of the things that shorten it. As a result, I will probably live twenty to twenty-five years longer than was expected for my birth group. In enabling me to live these added years, God has made possible something beyond raising the next generation and doing my share of the work. *Growing up*, then, means becoming free to do what God wants.

I must yet discover what God wants me to do as I continue *growing up*. That is where the church comes in. When I was baptized as an infant, the minister admonished the congregation to be my sponsor, my *godparents*, and to help my parents bring me up in such a way that, as I was *growing up*, I would choose to follow Christ's way and try to carry out God's will wherever I might be.

I still need that nurture from the church. As God's people, seeking to understand and carry out God's purpose on earth, I need their help in discerning how, in my later years, I am to be a part of God's scheme of things. As those who preserve and study the accumulated experience of God's activity among us, I need their encouragement as I try to learn whether I am called to new tasks that build on and continue my pilgrimage until now, or to ventures I cannot now even imagine.

In the chapters that follow I try to describe, for myself as much as for pastors and other church leaders, the dimensions of a pastoral ministry that nurtures women and men like me; people, who at midlife and beyond, are seeking to find their way through the unexpected and unplanned-for third of life that follows the completion of parenthood and career.

Chapter 2

A Time for Every Purpose

Everything that happens in this world happens at the time God chooses. He sets the time for birth and the time for death. . . .

— Ecclesiastes 3:1-2

Why do people grow old? A biologist might answer that aging is a characteristic of all living species. Growing older is a natural process that begins with birth and continues throughout life. A physician, on the other hand, might respond that aging is the consequence of living in a hazardous environment. Growing older is a gradual process of wear and tear resulting from illness, injuries and adverse living conditions. A demographer might say that aging is something that happens to societies when they become more affluent. There are fewer births, so the population gradually gets older. Fewer people die when they are young, so more live to be old. A sociologist might reply, instead, that aging is only a way of describing people that sometimes is useful. When there are more workers than jobs, for example, younger workers can be hired if older workers can be persuaded or required to quit working.

Such responses are helpful only if we are concerned with aging as a matter of curiosity or study. Such answers, however, are not likely to satisfy someone who wants to know why life moves inexorably from youth to age. Our hypothetical experts were dealing with such questions as: *What produces the symptoms commonly called aging? What causes people to age?* If we are concerned about growing older, we want to know instead, *Why must I live eighty or ninety years when fifty or sixty is enough to raise the next generation and achieve success at some career? What purpose is served by my growing older?*

Old age is not the most popular time of life. The popular senti-ment is that it is good to be young and bad to be old. This leads to discrimination against the old. We find it harder to get and keep jobs. We have to get along on less income. We are reminded often that we are less attractive than our younger neighbors and than we ourselves once were. If we try to stay young we discover it can't be done. One must grow old or die. Skin creams and hair darkeners, vitamins and exercise programs ultimately won't keep us from growing older. At best they make it more likely we will live long enough to become truly old.

Why *do* people grow old? What purpose does it serve? This book is about older people in the life of the church, so let's try a theologi-cal answer. Theology, once called the queen of the sciences, may provide a perspective other sciences overlook. We don't have a lot of space to devote to this, so let's not try a complete theological discussion of aging. Let's begin, rather, with a simple proposition: *People grow old because God means for them to do so.*

You may see this answer as unnecessarily complicating an al-ready unpleasant subject. Growing older is bad enough; why blame God for it? Surely a caring God would not wish upon beloved crea-tures such an outcome. Perhaps, yet if it is not God's intention that humans grow older, then either some divine plan has gone seriously astray, or else aging is somehow a consequence of human behavior. Neither of those lines of reasoning is likely to increase the popular-ity of old age. To say that people grow older because God means for them to do so, is simply to say that old age has some purpose in God's scheme of things.

HUMANS SERVE A USEFUL PURPOSE

Old age is inseparably part of life. There is no historical evidence of a time when it did not exist. There is no reason to conclude that old age is something added to life more recently; that it was not always part of human life. To ask what is the purpose of old age is to ask whether there is more to the purpose of life than we had perceived. Let's begin, therefore, with this assumption: *The pur-pose of old age is consistent with the purpose of human life.*

Individuals whose own purpose in living has been completed in rearing children and pursuing a career often live much longer than is required for those concerns. If their lives have a purpose beyond what they perceive, that purpose must somehow be attributed to whatever enables them to live so long. Some humans have always lived long lives. There is no reason, therefore, to assume that human effort alone has made long life possible, only that it has enabled more people to enjoy the possibility.

If long life is not the result of human effort, then we must posit some creator as its source. There is no empirical evidence that the universe was created. No maker can be deduced from careful observation. No search for a first cause, no discovery of some initial big bang, will lead us to a creating God. Nevertheless, Christians affirm that creation *has* a purpose, and that there *is* a being whose purpose it is. We believe that earth and its inhabitants are God's handiwork.

Creation's purpose is no more self-evident, however, than its maker. We will discover it neither by careful scrutiny of earth itself, nor by diligent search for earth's origins. We will learn God's purpose for our lives through neither self-understanding nor genealogy. Each life's purpose is determined by God, known to God, and will be revealed by God at the right time. How, then, are we to discover God's purpose for our life?

The biblical creation stories allude to God's purpose in particular creative acts. God makes humans so the earth will be under the control of beings like God, and makes grain and fruit so that animals and people will have food (Genesis 1:26-30). God makes a man to cultivate and guard the earth, then adds birds and animals, and finally a woman, so that the man will not be alone (Genesis 2:7-24). Each act reveals something of God's nature as creator, but falls short of revealing the purpose for creation itself.

God's purpose may be revealed more in what God says about creation than in the reasons given for specific creative acts. God is pleased with creation. Again and again, as it takes shape, God looks at the results and pronounces them good (Genesis 1:4-31). Creation's goodness could be equated simply with the innocence (Genesis 2:25) of Eden's residents before their disobedience and banishment. Because the earth's human occupants and guardians (Genesis 2:15) have turned to evil, fallen from grace, and are now under God's displeasure, we should then have to conclude that creation itself has been tainted by human failure and is no longer good in God's sight.

The account of the Flood (Genesis 6:1-9:17) suggests, however, that creation's goodness is not the simple equivalent of moral innocence. Discovering that earth's occupants have taken up evil ways, God regrets having made them and put them on earth. Yet their sin does not nullify God's original intent. God chooses to *renew* creation rather than destroy it. The earth itself, and a pair of each species, are saved from destruction. Human beings are also spared, but they are not restored to their original innocence. They are neither relieved of their responsibility to cultivate and guard the earth, nor spared the burden of toil and the pain of childbirth that have become their lot as a consequence of their disobedience (Genesis 3:16-19). That God chooses not to destroy creation suggests that its value, though compromised, has not been lost because of human evil.

Creation is initially good, of course, because God made it. Its goodness, however, may be more a matter of its nature than its initial state. Suppose God had never made a world before. God's initial response to the earth and its inhabitants may have been much like Alexander Graham Bell's reaction when his voice finally carried over the wire to Watson in the next room; "Eureka! It works! It does what I hoped it would do!" If such be the case, then creation is good simply because it is useful and serves God's purpose. That usefulness remains intact despite human failings. Humans are part of creation and therefore partake of its usefulness. They are good because they too are suited to God's original intent. Even when their ways and their thoughts differ from God's (Isaiah 55:8-9), they remain capable of carrying out God's purposes. This capacity to carry out God's purpose is at the very heart of our nature as we are part of God's creation. If we would understand how God's purpose applies to us, we must pay particular attention to what God says about the creation of humans.

HUMANS BEAR GOD'S LIKENESS

Humans do not resemble God in any discernible way, yet they are made in God's likeness (Genesis 1:26-27). Whatever God makes will, of course, bear the likeness of its maker; so it is with anything that someone makes. The idea that humans are made like

God is akin to the reality that each of us resembles our parents. When others look at us, they often see that likeness. If they have known our parents, they comment, "He's a chip off the old block; she's the image of her mother." The likeness to our parents is more than physical resemblance. Because we carry many of the same genes, we inherit some of their physical and mental capabilities. Living in close proximity to them for many years, we learn much of what they know and often adopt many of their values. Resembling them in so many ways, we reveal our parents to others, even to those who never knew them. More important, perhaps, we often carry on what they began, building on foundations they laid.

Such likeness to God is most clearly visible in one particular human, Jesus of Nazareth, who "has in himself the full nature of God" (Colossians 1:19). When Philip asked, "Lord, show us the Father"; Jesus replied, "Whoever has seen me has seen the Father" (John 14:8-9). What Jesus did with his life was "the deeds my Father gave me to do. . . . " (John 5:36). The image of God so clearly visible in Jesus is in us as well. More potential than reality, perhaps, it is nonetheless there. To say that we are made in God's image is, therefore, to say that we are capable of revealing God to others as children reveal their parents, and that we are capable of carrying forward God's work in the world as children carry on their parent's work.

To be made in God's image is to be called into covenant with God. When Abram was very old, God came to him and said, "I am the Almighty God. Obey me and always do what is right. I will make my covenant with you and give you many descendants. . . . You also must agree to keep the covenant with me, both you and your descendants in future generations" (Genesis 17:1-2, 9).

One obvious requirement of such a covenant is that we shall have to become parents. God's covenant is an "everlasting covenant" (Genesis 17:19). God's covenant provides for future relationships between creator and creation. Only if we bear and rear children will there be future generations to care for God's handiwork.

Such a covenant can only be possible if there is understanding between creature and creator. To be made in God's image is to be enough like God to share experiences, ideas and beliefs with God as though we spoke the same language. To have such fellowship with God is to know the need to respond to God's word. The rest of creation obeys the divine will without any conscious will of its own. Stars and planets follow their established courses, animals obey their instincts. As objects of God's self-revelation, however, we are capable of conscious choice. We can discern God's will, and either obey or disobey. We can perceive God's presence, and experience God's judgment. God requires humans to exercise this freedom with a responsibility not required of nature.[1]

Because we are made in God's image, we are capable of mistaking ourselves for God (Genesis 3:1-7). If we claim for ourselves God's attributes, such as knowledge of what is good and what is evil, we reveal only our folly and our nakedness (Genesis 3:7). God is revealed through us, not by our actions, but only by grace. Yet, if we believe that God is revealed in Jesus and that the work Christ does is God's work, we will do as much, and more (John 14:11-12).

To be made in God's image is to be made capable of eternal life. Whatever is created has a way of belonging forever to its maker. It can be sold, given away, crushed, broken, burned, yet exist forever in the mind of its creator. A child can grow to be someone far different than its parents had hoped or dreamed. It can be corrupt, evil, even dangerous, yet remain forever *their* child. We are neither independent nor free, but "derived from, and made for, God."[2] We belong forever to God. Though we turn from God again and again, God will not give us up; will not turn from us in anger; will not destroy us (Hosea 11:1-9). Nothing in all creation can separate us from God's eternal love (Romans 8:39).

HUMANS HAVE A PARTICULAR RESPONSIBILITY

Having made the heavens and the earth, and all that fills them, God created humans (Genesis 1:26-30), making them inferior only to their creator (Psalm 8:5). Though made in God's likeness, our powers are by no means comparable. We cannot guide the stars or command the day to dawn; we cannot make the lightening flash or the rain come down (Job 38:13-35). Yet God has given us dominion over creation (Genesis 1:28), and made us rulers over all that has been made (Psalm 8:6-8).

Having put humans in charge of creation, it may seem at first that God is finished with it. One need not take Genesis 1 too literally to believe that, having done it all in six days, God might have taken a day off and then gone on to other divine concerns without looking back. If that were so, then we would be in a situation much like youngsters let loose in a candy store. Acting on the assumption that earth and its contents are ours to do with as we see fit, we would soon have a tummy ache of cosmic proportions. Lacking any clarity of purpose to guide our actions, we would probably devour the earth, and ourselves with it.

Gazing skyward on a starry night, one is aware that God has put together a very large universe within which the earth is a very minor planet. Without denying that God can be powerfully everywhere at all times, one might assume that God has put humans in charge of the planet so as not to run the entire universe singlehandedly. We might conclude that we have been left in charge so that God can spend an eon or so looking after other parts of creation. If we were content to be only caretakers, we might soon find ourselves in the unenviable difficulty of the servant who hid his master's money in the ground and did not improve its value (Matthew 25:24-28). On the other hand, aware that we are made in God's likeness, and believing that we know what is best for creation (Genesis 3:5), we might try to improve on God's original design, and soon reduce earth's beauty to an ugly and scarred caricature. God's plan will involve work on our part. Creation is not self-maintaining. If we are to make use of the earth's capacity to produce food, we will have to cultivate and till it. The grain and fruit God has provided (Genesis 1:29, 2:9) will not long sustain life if we do not expend some effort caring for the soil.

Furthermore, creation is not only for the use of one generation. If those who come after us are to enjoy its bounty, we will have to manage its resources. We will have to protect its scarce and fragile treasures. By granting us dominion over creation, God calls us to be more than workers. We are to be responsible for the earth and the skies, and for all the creatures who inhabit them. We are to guard the earth (Genesis 2:15). This is far more than a call to responsible ecology. To have dominion over creation is to be accountable for *all* that God has made. By putting us "in charge of the fish, the birds, and all the wild animals" (Genesis 1:28), God calls us to work toward that peaceful kingdom in which wolves and sheep live together and little children look after them (Isaiah 11:6-9).

We cannot exercise dominion over God's creation except as creatures ourselves. We have not, however, been left to our own devices. Made in the likeness of God, we are capable of communion with God. We cannot disregard God's purposes for the rest of creation, nor can we stand apart from it. As God's day-by-day administrators, we are agents of God's will yet intimately part of God's creation. We are to use creation in accordance with God's purpose, yet understand that creation itself is the setting within which *we* are to grow into closer communion with God.

As Christians, we cannot ask why God created human beings without also asking why God became human in Jesus of Nazareth. The God who created the heavens and the earth is the same God revealed to us in Jesus Christ (John 1:1-18). There is no suggestion in scripture that God's intent in redeeming us is at odds with the Creator's purpose in creating us. Instead, "creation was condemned to lose its purpose" and now "waits with eager longing . . . to be set free from its slavery to decay and . . . share the glorious freedom of the children of God" (Romans 8:19-21). We must add a second assumption to our discussion: *The purpose of creation is consistent with the purpose of the incarnation.*

"God loved the world so much that he gave his only Son, so that everyone who believes in him may have eternal life" (John 3:16). In Jesus Christ, God's love is revealed and our answering love is called forth. To love God is to love and care for that which is God's, that is, the universe and all the beings who inhabit it. The Christian doctrine of creation is concerned particularly with human beings; it speaks of God's love for us and our ability to love each other.

To encounter God's love through Jesus Christ is to be called to become more fully human. When the disciples of John the Baptist asked Jesus if he were the one John had said was going to come, Jesus answered, "Go back and tell John what you are hearing and seeing: the blind can see, the lame can walk, those who suffer from dreaded skin diseases are made clean, the deaf hear, the dead are brought back to life, and the Good News is preached to the poor" (Matthew 11:3-5). In Jesus Christ, we meet the God who rules creation and determines all things. It is not our discovery, however, but God's revelation to us.

To have dominion over creation is to share in God's saving work, to be a coworker with Christ. To be in charge of creation is to be responsible for God's world and to minister in God's behalf. It is to be aware of what Christ is doing in the world, and to be doing it with him. It is to comprehend the message Marley delivered to Scrooge: "Mankind was my business. The common welfare was my business; charity, mercy, forbearance, and benevolence, were all my business. The dealings of my trade were but a drop of water in the comprehensive ocean of my business!"³ It is to enter into a covenant as old as Abraham and Moses and as new as Sister Theresa and Martin Luther King, Jr.

Older people are not excluded from this call. The ministry *of* older people to others is as important as others' ministry *to* older people. The God who gives life also gives the gifts needed for ministry. Our perception that older people need our help and our service must not keep us from understanding their worth, their potential, and their need to be in ministry to others:

> There are different kinds of spiritual gifts, but the same Spirit gives them. There are different ways of serving, but the same Lord is served. There are different abilities to perform service, but the same God gives ability to all for their particular service. The Spirit's presence is shown in some way in each person for the good of all. The Spirit gives one person a message full of wisdom, while to another person the same Spirit gives a message full of knowledge. One and the same Spirit gives faith to one person, while to another he gives the power to heal. The Spirit gives one person the power to work miracles; to another, the gift of speaking God's message; and to yet another, the ability to tell the difference between gifts that come from the Spirit and those that do not. To one person he gives the ability to speak in strange tongues, and to another he gives the ability to explain what is said. But it is one and the same Spirit who does all this; as he wishes, he gives a different gift to each person.
>
> —I Corinthians 12:4-11

God's gifts build up Christ's body, bringing people together in the unity of faith and knowledge, so that they "become mature people, reaching to the very height of Christ's full stature. . . . [They] shall no longer be children, . . . [but] grow up in every way to Christ, who is the head" (Ephesians 4:13-15). God's gifts become our ministry through Christ's redemption of human responsibility for God's creation. There is no indication that in old age God's gifts become less operative; no thought that those in later life are exempted or excluded from that ministry.

God's plan is for everyone. All, young, old and those in the middle, are included. The losses that accompany aging—the reduced income, the children growing up, the death of a spouse—can be a means of emptying oneself (Philippians 2:7) "of the distracting ambitions and false criteria of value that stand as obstacles to one's realization of the transcendent."⁴ They can be a means to learning the importance of *inter*dependendence, a human relationship of far greater consequence for believers and nonbelievers alike than the *in*dependence our society deems so important.

Growing older can have a purpose as much as does growing up. When we are young we can, and do, develop our own purposes for when we are *grown up*. Just so, as we grow older, we can develop new purposes for our lives. Whatever aims we pursue at any stage in life may, of course, not be at all in harmony with God's intentions. As we grow older, we are called, as when we were first growing up, to discover God's will for our lives, and make it our own.

IT'S ALL IN THE TIMING

If God means for us to grow old, we have only to wait for the passing of time. When God created the light and the darkness, and set the sun amid the one and the moon amid the other, time began (Genesis 1:14). If some purpose is to be served by growing older, we need only wait while the earth makes a few more trips around the sun. Time moves relentlessly onward, the hours becoming days, the days years, the years a lifetime. We can do nothing to hasten or retard its passing. "Everything that happens in the world happens at the time God chooses" (Ecclesiastes 3:1).

Time is commonly understood in terms of minutes, hours, days and years. They form an orderly succession of uniform compartments in which to store experiences. We keep track of family life and world events by means of clocks and calendars. They work because the universe is like a great clock. We regulate our lives to earth's rotation and its travel around the sun, and the moon's travel around the earth. Artificial light can make night into day, but we still rise, go about our affairs, and return to bed when our part of earth is toward the sun. Air conditioning can make summer into spring, but we operate our schools, choose our clothing, and schedule our vacations in rhythm with earth's four seasons.

Time influences our lives in many ways. Its cyclical nature is represented by the ancient symbol of *yin* and *yang*, in which two tear-drop shaped figures curved together form a circle. One half represents light, the sun, spring and summer; the other half dark, the moon, autumn and winter. As the circle rotates, it symbolizes the daily cycle of light and darkness and the annual cycle of four seasons. The endless repetition of the seasons is thought to be echoed in the endless repetition of human lives and events. "Whatever happens or can happen has already happened before. God makes the same thing happen again and again" (Ecclesiastes 3:15).

There are linear patterns as well. Time began with the creation of light and darkness, and will end when a new heaven and earth replace this heaven and earth (Revelation 21:1). In individual lives, time begins with birth and ends with death. It moves in only one direction and its passage is relentless and inescapable. Time is finite and limited and one's allotment is known only to God. Time is inexorably used up, and can, therefore, be wasted. Once a minute, a year, a lifetime has elapsed, there can be no going back. Sometime during middle age, our attitude toward time therefore begins to change. We become more keenly aware that God "sets the time for birth and the time for death . . ." (Ecclesiastes 3:2). We take up exercise, hoping to prolong the years that remain. We seek out new interests, wanting the final years to be better than our memories of the ones already passed.

The clocks that keep track of time have a way of running down. The theory of entropy holds that anything that runs gradually runs down. If that is true, the universe is slowly running down and the centrifugal force that holds the planets in their courses is slowly weakening so that eventually they will fall into the sun. Whether we believe that, we act as though human lives gradually run down. We liken the linear course of human life to a bell-shaped curve. We consider wrinkles and gray hair sure signs that one is slowing down. So powerful is this imagery that it functions as self-fulfilling prophecy. Expecting to slow down seems to induce physical decline when no other cause is apparent.

The perception that time and aging are inextricably linked leads us to think poorly of older people. We consider those past age 50 as on the downhill side of time's curve. We think twice about hiring them, view their experience as outmoded, and laugh when they describe themselves as still young. We assume time is running out for those past age 65. We encourage them to cease working and play in the little time they have left. We are quite sure those past 75 or 80 have nothing to contribute to society's well-being and little to pass on to future generations. We call astrology a harmless diversion and deny that the movement of stars and planets can influence human affairs, yet we act as though an individual has undergone radical change once the earth has gone around the sun a few more times.

We run from time rather than make the most of it. "Blind to the marvel of the present moment, we live with memories of moments misled, and in anxiety about an emptiness that lies ahead."[5] Time destroys what it has created, leaving us fearful of dying. Everything moves in an instant from not yet to no more. "Time is to us a sarcasm, a slick, treacherous monster with a jaw like a furnace incinerating every moment of our lives."[6] Fearing nothingness and nonbeing, we "try to realize the meaning of life within time."[7] Anxiety turns the future into a "sterile void" that we try to fill with "planning, predictions, reasonable expectations, insurance policies. . . . [so that] inertia prevents us from having a future and hangs on to *sameness*."[8]

Nonetheless, our lives are lived out within the framework provided by time. We cannot delay its passing even to pursue God's will a bit farther. Nor can we, when life's work is done or health has failed, will the speedy coming of the end. Time is beyond our control and old age is inevitable. However, as much as we trust that God's purposes are greater than our comprehension, we find it difficult to believe that God's purpose for old age is simply that we endure it. One more assumption is thus needed: *The purpose of old age is consistent with the nature of time.*

Our discomfort about time arises not so much from the boundaries it creates as from a too limited conception of time itself. In the New Testament, two common Greek words are the root translation of the English word *time*. One, *chronos*, has to do with the flow of time as described above. The other, *kairos*, has to do with moments of time in which something significant happens. *Chronos* is time as we experience it in nature, *kairos* is time as we encounter it in history. *Chronos* is time as a measurable quantity, while *kairos* is time as a favorable or decisive event.

As *chronos*, time is an aspect of our creatureliness. Its relentless progress is a given. We can no more alter the flow of time than we can make the sun come up in the west. God set the earth spinning in a course around the sun, but humans invented clocks and calendars and decided that 65 years is as long as one life can be useful. From time as *chronos* we derive a chronological view of aging that is the basis of most of the age bias, stereotyping and discrimination common to our society. From the perspective of *chronos*, the elderly can have little social value because they have little or no time left.

As *kairos*, time is an aspect of our creation in God's image and of our responsibility to care for everything that God has made. Here the issue is not how much or how little time there is, but what we make of the time we have. *Kairos* supports both a functional and a social understanding of aging because it affirms both our capacity for communion with God and each other and our opportunity and call to use every moment to carry on God's saving work. From the perspective of *kairos*, the elderly have value comparable to others. Older adults are capable of encounters with God and able to do God's will. It is not the lateness of the hour (II Samuel 19:34) that matters, but the opportunity of the moment (Joshua 14:12).

In first century Greek usage, *kairos* connotes something akin to the English word *timing*. Where *chronos* is clock time, *kairos* is auspicious time. Thus John the Baptist proclaimed: "The right time has come, . . . and the Kingdom of God is near! Turn away from your sins and believe the Good News!" (Mark 1:15). Another time, Jesus said to his disciples: "You go on to the festival. I am not going to this festival, because the right time has not come for me" (John 7:8). It was the right time for the disciples to go to Jerusalem to worship, but not yet the right time for Jesus to go there to die.

As every moment is *chronos*, a unit of clock time, so every moment is potentially *kairos*, the right time for something to happen.

In every life there are particular moments of *kairos* time. Events such as birth, puberty, marriage and death are marked by liturgical rites such as baptism, confirmation, wedding and funeral, because we have learned that God confronts us in these events. But there are other moments of *kairos*. We meet a stranger or fall in love, we marry or divorce, a child is born or a parent dies, we enter school or graduate, we get our first job or retire. In any or all of these and thousands of other events we may encounter God. " 'When, Lord, did we ever see you hungry and feed you, or thirsty and give you drink? When did we ever see you a stranger and welcome you in our homes, or naked and clothe you? When did we ever see you sick or in prison, and visit you?' The King will reply, 'I tell you, whenever you did this for [someone] . . . , you did it for me!' " (Matthew 25:37-40).

There is one event of *kairos* time, however, which is particularly significant for all humans. It is the moment of redemption, the central event of human history. How can Christ's death 2000 years ago, halfway around the world, affect us? If we view the Christ event as something that occurred in *chronos* time, the question is inevitable. To answer it, we might need to determine just where and when Jesus of Nazareth lived and died, then trace a chronology of cause and effect from Jesus' atoning death to that moment in our own passage from birth to death when we first comprehended our salvation. If instead we view the Christ event as a moment in *kairos* time, the question badly misses the mark. *Kairos* time is "fulfilled time."[9] In Christ's death and resurrection all of human history, including our particular history, is fulfilled. Christ's saving act is an encounter with God in which *we* are chosen, elected, called. The purpose of creation becomes our purpose in the here and now. In the same way, God encountered our parents, the sixteenth century reformers, Saul on the way to Damascus, and Sarai and Abram.

God is said to be eternal, timeless, the Alpha (beginning) and the Omega (ending). Christ is said to be the same yesterday, today and forever. Concepts such as beginning and ending, past, present and future, are derived from an understanding of time as *chronos*. So understood, time devalues the old as those near the ending, those with no future. God encounters us in time as *kairos* (event, happening, present moment). In *kairos* time, our age, defined by *chronos* time, becomes irrelevant. The tales of Israel's founders (see Chapter 3) make clear that age was no deterrent in their response to God's call or to Israel's need. It is not how many, or how few, years we have lived that matters, but our readiness to hear and answer God's call.

Considered as *chronos*, creation occurred at the beginning of time; considered as *kairos*, creation is an ongoing phenomenon. Our experience confirms the latter view. The execution of a painting or the composition of a concerto is a work of creation. What matters is not the amount of time needed for their completion, nor the precise moment in which they were begun or finished, but the human milieu out of which they sprang and which were transformed by their existence. A painting is not a masterpiece because of the number of hours or days required to complete it, but because of the interaction that occurs between the viewer, the canvas and oils, and the artist. A concerto is not a masterpiece because of the age of its composer, but because of the interaction that takes place between the listener, the musician and the composer. Because they occur in *kairos* time rather than *chronos* time, such encounters are not limited to the lifetime of the composer or the painter. Their works are timeless. Because they exist in *kairos* time, the age of the viewer or the listener is irrelevant as well. One moment is as good as another for the artist's work to be recreated in us. Whether that happens is determined not by the hands on the clock or the numbers on the calendar page, but by our readiness for it to happen.

Just so, God's redemptive event is timeless. It does not matter that Christ's death occurred 2000 years ago, halfway round the world. It is God's action that turns a particular date into an event that in turn implements God's purpose for creation. Such events form a "redemptive history." The believer participates in this history in the "present" by sharing in events that occurred in the "past" and partaking of God's promises for the "future."[10] Because Christ's redemptive act occurs in *kairos* time rather than *chronos* time, such encounters are not limited to Christ's "lifetime." They are "timeless." Because they occur in *kairos* time, our age is irrelevant. One moment is as good as another for our redemption.

If we understand time only as *chronos*, we are likely to approach old age with dread. We will always be wondering if today the clock will strike for the last time. What will it matter that God has a purpose for old age? That we are made in God's image? That we are capable of carrying forward God's saving work? If nothing we do can alter time's progress, why should we expect our actions to change anything else in creation?

If we understand that time is also *kairos*, we can approach old age with anticipation. We can be eager to see how God will yet work out creation's purpose through us. We can perceive new opportunities to experience God's presence and to share with others God's Good News as once it was shared with us. We can begin each new day ready for whatever surprises it may hold.

People grow old because growing old is part of human life as God makes it. God's image does not fade with the passing years. One can love and care for what God has made at any age. God's call is to all people. It matters not how young or old we are, only whether we are ready to answer God's call.

NOTES

1. Emil Brunner, THE CHRISTIAN DOCTRINE OF CREATION AND REDEMPTION [DOGMATICS, VOL. II] (Philadelphia: Westminster Press, 1952) 55-57.

2. Brunner, DOGMATICS, II, 55.

3. Charles Dickens, A CHRISTMAS CAROL.

4. Evelyn Eaton Whitehead, "Religious Images of Aging: An Examination of Themes in Contemporary Religious Thought" in Carol LeFevre and Perry Le-Fevre (Eds.), AGING AND THE HUMAN SPIRIT: A READER IN RELIGION AND GERONTOLOGY (Chicago: Exploration Press, 1981), 63.

5. Rabbi Abraham J. Heschel, "The Older Person and the Family in the Perspective of Jewish Tradition" in AGING AND THE HUMAN SPIRIT, 41.

6. *Ibid.*

7. Brunner, FAITH, HOPE, AND LOVE (Philadelphia: Westminster Press, 1956), 53.

8. Frederick S. Perls, IN AND OUT THE GARBAGE PAIL (New York: Bantam Books, 1972), 174.

9. Paul Tillich, "Kairos" in A HANDBOOK OF CHRISTIAN THEOLOGY (Cleveland: Meridian Books, 1958), 195.

10. Oscar Cullman, CHRIST AND TIME (Philadelphia: Westminster Press, 1950), 76.

Chapter 3

Heroes, Heroines and Role Models

> Then the Lord asked Abraham, "Why did Sarah laugh and
> say, 'Can I really have a child when I am so old?' Is anything
> too hard for the Lord? As I said, nine months from now I will
> return, and Sarah will have a son."
>
> —Genesis 18:13-14

When we were young, those who were older became our heroes,
heroines and role models. As we developed our agendas for growing up, they were our examples of what we could become. Some,
only a year or so older, showed us how to manage future stages of
growing up. Others showed us how to be parents, or how to do
different kinds of work.

As we move into our later years, we need new heroes, heroines
and role models to show us how it can be in the years that lie ahead.
They must be examples of what to do when children are grown and
careers have ended. They must show us how to care for our parents
when they can no longer care for themselves, and how to face the
infirmity that may be our lot in the last days or years of our lives.
Most of all, they must help us discover what God calls us to when
the basic tasks of adult life have been completed.

In the Bible are the stories of older women and men which can
teach us much of what we need to know about growing up. More
important, they can show us how to discern what God has in mind
for our later years.

Life was shorter for most people in biblical times than in our day,
but old age was far from unknown. Biblical writers made note of
the ages of the people about whom they wrote. Their tales of those
who lived long lives reveal that growing old in ancient times was a

lot like growing old today. Their admonitions about old age, along with some of the regulations they preserved, make clear that attitudes toward old age have not changed much from that day to this.

LIVING A LONG TIME

From the biblical point of view, to live long is normal, to die young is the exception (Genesis 6:3, Isaiah 65:20). Still, we are reluctant to believe that, generation after generation, people in ancient times could have lived the very long lives recorded in Scripture. We know that their stories were part of Israel's oral tradition for centuries before they were finally written down. We are likely to believe therefore that their ages have been exaggerated in the repeated telling of Israel's history. We are sure this must be so when we read that Adam lived 930 years, his son Seth 912 years, his grandson Enosh 905 years, and that Shem, Ham and Japeth, were born after their father Noah was 500 years old (Genesis 5:3-32).

The people of ancient Israel probably lived an average of no more than twenty-five years. Still some of Israel's leaders are reported to have lived very long lives. Some will take literally their reported ages, others will suspect that they are folk history. In either case, it is clear that some people lived longer than average lives and undertook important tasks quite late in life. Sarah was 127 years old when she died (Genesis 23:1), but Abraham lived to be 175 (Genesis 25:7-8), and their son Isaac died when 180 years old (Genesis 35:29). Moses lived 120 years, and when he died "he was as strong as ever, and his eyesight was still good" (Deuteronomy 34:7). Jacob lived to be 147 years old (Genesis 47:28); both Joseph (Genesis 50:22) and Joshua (Joshua 24:29) lived to the age of 110 years.

Others too are said to have lived very long lives. Aaron died at 123 (Numbers 33:38-39), and Eli died at 99 after having been a leader in Israel for 40 years (I Samuel 4:12-18). Jehoida, high priest during the reign of Joash, lived to be 130 (II Chronicles 24:15). Job lived 140 years after his family and fortune were restored to him (Job 42:16-17). After rescuing her city from Holofernes by first beguiling then decapitating him, Judith lived to be 105 (Judith 16:23).

Few people lived very long in ancient times because virulent disease so often ended life very early. Less than a century ago one of every five deaths in the United States was a child under one year and one of three deaths was a child under age fifteen. Yet if a child born a hundred years ago survived childhood, sixty or seventy years became likely and eighty or ninety would not have been impossible. That must also have been the case in ancient Israel, which knew far less about nutrition, sanitation and disease than we did a century ago. If one survived childhood in ancient Israel, the chances of living to a ripe old age must have been considerably enhanced.

Even so, it seems unlikely that anyone could have lived as long as some are said to have done. Yet some of Israel's ancient leaders apparently did live very long lives. They survived for long years in an environment that was, at best, hazardous and demanding. Was there something special about them? Did they possess some special knowledge or magic that warded off evil and protected them against harm? Or were they natural survivors, endowed with genes favoring long life and fortunate enough to escape the diseases that carried away some of their peers and the battles that destroyed others?

Older people are sometimes thought to have lived long because they are wise. This is evident in the deference with which younger people sometimes treat their elders, out of respect for their greater experience:

> I am young, and you are old,
>   so I was afraid to tell you what I think.
> I told myself that you ought to speak,
>   that you older men should share your wisdom.

> —Job 32:6-7

But old age does not necessarily bring wisdom. Rather:

> . . . it is the spirit of the Almighty God
> that comes to men and gives them wisdom.
> It is not growing old that makes them wise
> or helps them to know what is right.

> —Job 32:8-9

For human wisdom always falls short of God's greater wisdom:

> Old men have wisdom,
> but God has wisdom and power.
> Old men have insight;
> but God has insight and power to act.
>
> —Job 12:12

Could the long lives of Israel's ancient leaders have something to do instead with their response to God's call? Long life is sometimes attributed to righteousness. "Long life is the reward of the righteous; grey hair is a glorious crown" (Proverbs 16:31). "Happy is the person whom God corrects! . . . Like wheat that ripens till harvest time, [he] will live to a ripe old age" (Job 5:17, 26). The righteous "are like trees planted in the house of the Lord, that flourish in the Temple of our God, that still bear fruit in old age and are always green and strong" (Psalm 92:13-14).

BEING IN COVENANT WITH GOD

Long life is the lot of the *righteous*. The righteous are those who are obedient to God's commandments. Their obedience is grounded in faithful study of the Law:

> Happy are those
>   who reject the advice of evil men,
>   who do not follow the example of sinners
>   or join those who have no use for God.
> Instead, they find joy in obeying the Law of the Lord,
>   and they study it day and night.
> They are like trees that grow beside a stream,
>   that bear fruit at the right time,
>   and whose leaves do not dry up.
> They succeed in everything they do.
>
> —Psalm 1:1-3

The righteous are also those who maintain the integrity and wholeness of the family, the community, and the nation. Long life is promised to those who respect their parents (Exodus 20:12, Deuteronomy 5:16); those who refrain from speaking evil and work for peace (Psalm 34:12-14); and those who are fair and just (Deuteronomy 16:20). Righteousness involves more than simply following orders. Essentially, it is a matter of being in a covenant relationship with God.

God made a covenant with Abraham when the latter was 99 years old. He was promised that faithfully keeping the covenant would bring long life (Genesis 15:15). "I will be your God and the God of your descendants. . . . You also must agree to keep the covenant with me, both you and your descendants in future generations" (Genesis 17:7-8). Moses was assured that those who followed Yahweh's laws would live, while those who followed the ways of the Egyptians or the Canaanites would die (Leviticus 18:3-5, Deuteronomy 30:16-20).

Initially, it seems, we were meant to live forever. The first humans were told to eat fruit from the tree that gives life and from any other tree in the garden *except* the one that gives knowledge of what is good and what is bad (Genesis 2:9-17). When they disobeyed and ate the fruit of that tree, they were sent out of the garden forever, so that they could no longer eat fruit from the tree that gives life (Genesis 3:22-24). What is important about Adam's descendants, therefore, is not that they lived hundreds of years, but that each finally died. Whether their deaths were direct punishment for their sin, or the natural consequences of the hard work, the pain of childbirth, and the enmity with nature to which they were condemned (Genesis 3:17-19), they died.

Eons later, angered over the evil ways of his creatures, God established limits for all human life. "I will not allow people to live forever; they are mortal. From now on they will live no longer than 120 years" (Genesis 6:3). The apocryphal Book of Jubilees measures lives in fifty-year *jubilees*.[1] From Creation to the Flood, individual lives averaged nineteen jubilees (950 years); after that, because of human evil, anyone who lived a jubilee and a half (75 years) was accounted as old, and before they had lived two jubilees (100 years), knowledge would forsake them (Jubilees 23:9-12).

According to scripture, an early death is the lot of the *unrighteous*. "Our life," writes the Psalmist, "is cut short by your anger;

it fades away like a whisper" (Psalm 90:9). Unrighteousness is not understood as simply wrongdoing or disobedience; rather, it is the opposite of being in covenant with God. Adam and Eve were warned not to eat the fruit of the tree that gives knowledge of what is good and what is bad. When they did, they broke covenant with God. Thus separated from God, they eventually died (Genesis 2:16-17). Achan disobeyed the order to destroy everything in Jericho and kept some things for himself. Having set himself outside the covenant between God and Israel, he died (Joshua 7:25). Eli's sons contemptuously disregarded that same covenant, and God promised Eli, "no one in your family will ever again live to be old" (I Samuel 2:32). When Ananias and Sapphira kept back part of their property and did not put all they had into the common pot, they denied the covenant between God and the new Church and they died (Acts 5:1-10).

Death is not, however, seen as simply punishment for wrongdoing. It is rather the natural consequence of unrighteousness, of a broken covenant relationship with God. Unfortunately, the same word, *death*, denotes for us both the last event in our temporal life (physical death) and a permanent condition of isolation from God (spiritual death). It is the latter that scripture sees as the natural consequence of avoiding the covenant God holds out to us. Spiritual death is far more to be feared than the physical death we all must encounter. God's mercy, however, is greater than our sin of avoidance. His love for us is so powerful that even our state of spiritual death can be transformed into eternal life in Christ (Ephesians 2:4-5).

The long life the Bible promises to the righteous is *eternal life* rather than long years of temporal life. In place of this temporal and moribund life, "God has given us eternal life, and this life has its source in his Son" (I John 5:11). With such assurance, we can wish with Paul "to leave this life and be with Christ. . . . " (Philippians 1:23). In breaking covenant with God, Adam and Eve, Achan, Hophni and Phinehas, Ananias and Sapphira each broke their vital connection to the ground of being, the very source of life. Eternal life comes from God, not through trees in a garden, but through a covenant relationship. *In covenant with God we live; apart from God we die.*

A few people have always lived extraordinarily long lives. Scholars today estimate that, biologically, humans have a potential life *span* of 120 years. Modern medical science has extended average life *expectancy* by eliminating some of the causes of early death and controlling others. Nonetheless, disease, accidents, war, and adverse living conditions still shorten life for most people. These manifestations of human sin and evil reveal how broken is our covenant with God. In the beginning, God created humans and instructed them to bear many children so that their descendants would live all over the earth and bring it under their control. "I am putting you in charge of the fish, the birds, and all the wild animals" (Genesis 1:28). "Then the Lord God placed the [human beings] in the Garden of Eden to cultivate it and guard it" (Genesis 2:15).

Adam and Eve broke the covenant with God, but it was later renewed with Abraham and his descendants (Genesis 15:1-21, 7:1-27), and again with Moses and the people of Israel (Exodus 24:1-18). In Jesus Christ, God once again offers to covenant with us (Matthew 26:27, Mark 14:24, Luke 22:20, I Corinthians 11:25). If we live in covenant with God, our days will be long. "I am an old man now; I have lived a long time, but I have never seen a good man abandoned by the Lord. . . . " (Psalm 37:25). If we break or reject God's covenant, we will die. "Death is the destiny of all the wicked, of all those who reject God" (Psalm 9:17).

LIVING ISN'T EASY

Long or short, life is not always easy. The advancing years sometimes bring physical problems. Isaac, Jacob, Eli and Ahijah all suffered blindness or failing vision in late life (Genesis 27:1, 48:10, I Samuel 3:2, 4:15, I Kings 14:4). Barzillai was hard of hearing and unable to taste his food (II Samuel 19:35). David suffered chills (I Kings 1:1-4), and Asa had problems with his feet or was impotent (I Kings 15:23).[2]

Because those who are growing older do sometimes experience chronic illness, loss of memory and other physical ailments, stereotypes often develop around the commonly perceived attributes of old age. It is clear from the Scriptures that this was as true in biblical times as it is today. By the writing of the Psalms, the expectation of long life had been replaced by a different view. "Seventy years is all we have—eighty years, if we are strong; yet all they bring us is trouble and sorrow; life is soon over, and we are gone" (Psalm 90:10). Injunctions to honor one's parents (Exodus 20:12, Proverbs 23:22), and respect the elderly (Leviticus 19:32, Proverbs 20:29), were probably needed reminders that respect and honor were not always accorded the old.

Compared to our own times, relatively few people lived past age fifty, yet the socially accepted view of old age seems to have been about the same in biblical times as now. Levites were to retire from active fulltime service in the Tabernacle at age fifty (Numbers 8:24-26). The fee to be paid to the priests for release from a religious vow was lower for those over age sixty (Leviticus 27:3-7). This may be an acknowledgement that older people were more likely to be poor (Leviticus 27:8); it certainly reflects a common attitude toward the circumstances of old age.

Among the popular stereotypes in our own day are those that imply a loss of sexual capacity as one grows older. Similar attitudes are reflected in the Scriptures. Abraham was amused and Zechariah incredulous at the suggestion of fathering a child in old age (Genesis 17:17, Luke 1:18). Sarah had long since completed menopause, so when a stranger announced she would bear a child in nine months, she laughed aloud and said, "Now that I am old and worn out, can I still enjoy sex? And besides, my husband is old too" (Genesis 18:12). When Paul wrote Titus to admonish older men to be "sober, sensible and self-controlled," and encourage older women to "behave as women should who live a holy life. . . ." (Titus 2:2-3), he probably reflected the popular belief that sexual activity is inappropriate, if not impossible, in later life. Apparently believing older women to be incapable of sexual desire, he warned Timothy not to "add any widow to the list of widows unless she is over sixty years of age." Younger widows' desires, he wrote, would make them want to marry again, thus breaking their vows to Christ (I Timothy 5:9-12).

One writer left behind as dismal a view of old age as any written in our own day:

So remember your Creator while you are still young, before those dismal days and years come when you will say, "I don't enjoy life." That is when the light of the sun, the moon, and the stars will grow dim for you, and the rain clouds will never pass away. Then your arms, that have protected you, will tremble, and your legs, now strong, will grow weak. Your teeth will be too few to chew your food, and your eyes too dim to see clearly. Your ears will be deaf to the noise of the street. You will barely be able to hear the mill as it grinds or music as it plays, but even the song of a bird will wake you from sleep. You will be afraid of high places, and walking will be dangerous. Your hair will turn white; you will hardly be able to drag yourself along, and all desire will be gone.

—Ecclesiastes 12:1-5

Almost everyone experiences some changes as they grow older, but it is seldom as bad as that.

Christians believe the Bible contains the revealed Word of God. We may therefore be uncertain about how to separate the inspired teachings of the Holy Spirit from the vestiges of popular social stereotypes, when we find both side by side in its pages. It is particularly a problem when the stereotypes of that day are similar to those of our own. We will be inclined to accord those stereotypes the credibility of inspired teaching rather than recognize them for what they are.

Today's religious leaders, even those deeply committed to equal treatment of women and members of racial and ethnic minorities, and to an inclusive church and society, sometimes find it difficult to be rid of deeply engrained stereotypes that are demeaning to others. Ageism pervades both church and society in our own day; we should not be surprised to find it present in the religious leaders of ancient Israel. Stereotypes that invoke discrimination against any group within society are a serious social problem, no matter how ancient they may be.

Not discounting the difficulties some experience in old age, stereotypes are often far from the truth. However, because they create expectations, they can powerfully influence the aging process.

From early childhood onward, our own aging is shaped by our perceptions of the older people around us. We seldom see them as they are, however. Instead, we filter what we see through the myths and images of aging that surround us. So powerful are these influences that older people often interpret what they see in themselves so that it fits the stereotypes they learned through the years. The cycle of discrimination is self-perpetuating and vicious.

Two men, both in their eighties, viewed their own aging quite differently. Barzillai, a rich man, had supplied David's troops with food during the final struggle with Absalom. When David invited Barzillai to return to Jerusalem with him, he replied: "I am already eighty years old, and nothing gives me pleasure any more. I can't taste what I eat and drink, and I can't hear the voices of singers. I would only be a burden to Your Majesty. I don't deserve such a great reward . . ." (II Samuel 19:35-36).

At forty, Caleb had been sent by Moses to spy out the land of Canaan; at eighty-five, he claimed from Joshua the land Moses had promised him forty-five years earlier (Numbers 14:24).

> Look at me! I am eighty-five years old and am just as strong today as I was when Moses sent me out. I am still strong enough for war or for anything else. Now then, give me the hill country that the Lord promised me on that day when my men and I reported. We told you then that the race of giants called the Anakim were there in large walled cities. Maybe the Lord will be with me, and I will drive them out, just as the Lord said."
>
> —Joshua 14:10-12

At any age, preoccupation with life's troubles makes them loom larger in our minds. If the present circumstances seem likely to overwhelm, it is little use to recite, "I cried because I had no shoes until I met a man who had no feet." It changes nothing that some are much worse off and others surmount difficulties like our own. It is easy to dwell on the problems of old age. Throughout life we are schooled to believe that it is bad to be old and good to be young. We can picture ourselves victims of circumstances beyond our control and pity ourselves for having grown old. Or we can stride confidently into old age determined to drive whatever giants there may be out of the hills God has promised us. The choice is ours. If we look for creative ways to make use of our later years, we will be going against the prevailing attitudes toward old age. We will succeed if we are certain that a different course lies open to us.

FACING UNCERTAINTY

People often fear old age, and go to great lengths to avoid its approach. Some fear death and the knowledge that the older they grow the more certain it becomes.

> We are going to our final resting place, and then there will be mourning in the streets. The silver chain will snap, and the golden lamp will fall and break; the rope at the well will break, and the water jar will be shattered. Our bodies will return to the dust of the earth, and the breath of life will go back to God, who gave it to us.
>
> — Ecclesiastes 12:5-7

No one can get out of this life alive. There is no way to avoid death. There is no potion we can drink, no security we can purchase, that will prevent its coming. Excessive preoccupation with its inevitability may, however, make us miss the creative possibilities in life. Jesus promises that those in covenant with God, through Christ himself, will never die for they have already passed from death to life (John 5:24, 8:51). Paul urges us to think of ourselves as already dead, yet alive because we are in covenant with God through Jesus Christ (Romans 6:11). Jesus assures us, "There are many rooms in my Father's house, and I am going to prepare a place for you, I would not tell you this if it were not so" (John 14:2). This temporal life must end in death. We cannot escape that. But we shall escape, we have already escaped, the more fearsome death of spiritual isolation from God forever.

More than death, older people often fear becoming dependent on others or being left alone. By the sea of Galilee, soon after his resurrection, Jesus spoke to Peter about growing old.

I tell you most solemnly,
when you were young
you put on your own belt
and walked where you liked;
but when you grow old
you will stretch out your hands,
and somebody else will put a belt round you
and take you where you would rather not go.

—John 21:18, Jerusalem Bible

When Jacob's sons had been to Egypt and seen their long lost and unrecognized brother Joseph, they returned to their father and told him they must take Benjamin, the youngest, back to Egypt with them. But Jacob said, "My son cannot go with you; his brother is dead, and he is the only one left. Something might happen to him on the way. I am an old man, and the sorrow you would cause me would kill me" (Genesis 42:38).

In the Psalms we find one of the most poignant expressions of the fear of being old and alone:

I have relied on you all my life;
   you have protected me since the day I was born.
My life has been an example to many,
   because you have been my strong defender.
All day long I praise you
   and proclaim your glory.
Do not reject me now that I am old;
   do not abandon me now that I am feeble.
You have taught me ever since I was young,
   and I still tell of your wonderful acts.
Now that I am old and my hair is gray,
   do not abandon me, O God!

—Psalm 71:6-9, 17-18

If we have faith, that is, if we are in covenant with God, we are never alone, in old age or at any other time.

Listen to me descendants of Jacob,
    all who are left of my people.
I have cared for you from the time you were born.
I am your God and will take care of you
    until you are old and your hair is gray.
I made you and will care for you;
    I will give you help and rescue you.

—Isaiah 46:3-4

God says, "I will save those who love me
    and will protect those who acknowledge me as Lord.
When they call to me, I will answer them;
    when they are in trouble, I will be with them.
    I will rescue them and honor them.
I will reward them with long life;
    I will save them."

—Psalm 91:14-16

More than obedience or social responsibility, righteousness is characterized by faith. It is that openness to love which makes it possible for God to covenant with us. It is that trust in God's intentions that is greater than our fears. Faith is the essential ingredient if we are to make the most of our later years.

It was faith that made Abraham able to become a father, even though he was too old and Sarah herself could not have children. He trusted God to keep his promise. Though Abraham was practically dead, from this one man came as many descendents as there are stars in the sky, as many as the numberless grains of sand on the seashore.

—Hebrews 11:11-12

Though she laughed at the idea (Genesis 18:12), Sarah surely needed a good deal of faith to get through nine months of pregnancy when she was very old.

How often the old are harbingers of the new things God is doing. At first, Zechariah would not believe the angel who told him that he and his wife Elizabeth would bear a child in their old age and would name him John. But when the child was born, Zechariah voiced a prayer (Luke 1:68-79) that recites God's acts of mercy to Israel and proclaims the redemption to come. As the *Benedictus*, it is recited daily in the office of Morning Prayer. It was faith that led both Simeon and Anna to the Temple on the day that Joseph and Mary came to present the newborn Messiah before the Lord (Luke 2:22-38). Simeon's prayer, the *Nunc Dimittis* (Luke 2:29-32), also speaks of the redemption to come.

Those who love God need not fear old age nor miss the promise held out to those who trust God. Long life will be restored in the new heaven and new earth which God is making. "Once again old men and women, so old that they use canes when they walk, will be sitting in the city squares" (Zechariah 8:4). "There will be no weeping there, no calling for help. Babies will no longer die in infancy, and all people will live out their life span. Those who live to be a hundred will be considered young" (Isaiah 65:19-20). When God pours out his spirit on everyone, "your old men will have dreams, and your young men will see visions" (Joel 2:28).

SAYING "YES" TO GOD'S CALL

Many of those whose long lives the Old Testament carefully records are remembered because they were leaders in Israel during times of difficulty and transition. What we should note in particular is that they were already advanced in years when their most significant leadership began. Abraham (then Abram) was 75 years old when he set out with his people for the land of Canaan (Genesis 12:4). Moses was 80 years old when he returned to Egypt to lead Israel out of slavery (Exodus 7:7). Joshua was about 80 years old when he succeeded Moses and led Israel across the Jordan (Joshua 1:1-2).[3]

Each had already done much before beginning that for which he is best remembered. Abram had already become a wealthy slaveholder and was old enough to have an adult nephew when he left Haran (Genesis 12:5). Moses had grown up as a prince in Egypt (Exodus 2:11), had married, and raised a family in Midian (Exodus 2:21-22), when God spoke to him from the burning bush. Joshua was already an adult when Moses first sent spies into Canaan (Numbers 13:8,16), then spent forty years in exile with Israel (Deuteronomy 2:7).

While the exact numbers of their years may be somewhat less than those recorded, there can be little doubt that these ancient leaders lived long lives. Moreover, they were lives filled with challenge and struggle. They led Israel through major transitions that affected them personally and significantly altered the course of Israel's history. Though already advanced in years, their age presented no barrier to God or their nation. Their long lives were exceptional but their leadership was not. Their wisdom, strength and righteousness came from God rather than from longevity.

Why, when times are critical in a community or in a nation, do some emerge as leaders while others do not? Why was it these individuals, and not others, who came forward when there was need in Israel for strong leadership?

Max Weber described three types of leadership: traditional, rational-legal, and charismatic.[4] Traditional leaders are those whose authority and power derive from social or economic status. By reason of birth or financial success, they are able to exercise influence over large numbers of people, sometimes whole nations or empires. The power and authority of rational-legal leaders is conferred on them by the decisions of others. Through election or appointment, they acquire control or influence over others. Charismatic leaders come into being through the call of a divine being in whom both leader and followers believe. Their leadership is largely the ability to influence others within a movement for change that is in itself compelling.

Abram began as a traditional leader, a rich man with slaves and flocks (Genesis 12:5, 13:2). So did Jacob, who had two wives (Genesis 29:15-30), and was very wealthy, with many flocks, slaves, camels and donkeys (Genesis 30:43). Joseph, on the other hand, became a rational-legal leader when appointed by Pharoah to virtually absolute power and authority over Egypt (Genesis 41:40-44).

Moses lacked similar foundations for the role he undertook. Though raised a prince in Egypt (Exodus 2:1-10), he had been 40 years in exile, a dependent of his father-in-law Jethro. He knew himself to be no longer a traditional leader. ''I am nobody. How can I go to the king and bring the Israelites out of Egypt?'' (Exodus 3:11). Though he later clearly displayed charismatic qualities, Moses at first doubted his capacity for leadership. Hesitant about speaking up before a powerful monarch, he said to God, "I have never been a good speaker, and I haven't become one since you began to speak to me. I am a poor speaker, slow and hesitant'' (Exodus 4:10).

Others had similar doubts. Before the presence of God, Isaiah cried out, "There is no hope for me! I am doomed because every word that passes my lips is sinful, and I live among a people whose every word is sinful'' (Isaiah 6:5). Jeremiah thought his *age* might be a problem. "I don't know how to speak; I am too young" (Jeremiah 1:6).

God does not choose people for leadership because they are already leaders.

> Now remember what you were . . . when God called you. From the human point of view few of you were wise or powerful or of high standing. God purposely chose what the world considers nonsense in order to shame the wise, and he chose what the world considers weak in order to shame the powerful. He chose what the world looks down on and despises and thinks is nothing, in order to destroy what the world thinks is important.
>
> —I Corinthians 1:26-28

Weber's description of charismatic leadership best fits those who stand out in Scripture. They came to leadership through the call of the God in whom they and their people believed. It did not matter whether they had wealth or power. Their ability to influence others lay in their divine call and in the movements they led. God called Abram, "Leave your country, your relatives, and your father's home, and go to a land that I am going to show you. I will give you many descendants and they will become a great nation'' (Genesis 12:1-2). God spoke to Moses from a bush that burned but was not consumed. "I have indeed heard the cry of my people, and I see how the Egyptians are oppressing them, Now I am sending you to the king of Egypt so that you can lead my people out of his country" (Exodus 3:9-10). After Moses' death, God spoke to Joshua, "Get ready now, you and all the people of Israel, and cross the Jordan River into the land I am giving them" (Joshua 1:2).

It surely is not God's intention that in old age all should become national leaders on the order of Moses or Joshua. Nor is it likely that God expects very many to become parents when they are 100 years old. It should be quite clear, nonetheless, that God does not regard advanced age as a handicap.

Some will be inclined to cast aside the evidence provided in Scripture. "Things were different then," they will say. Others will protest that Sarah and Abraham, along with a number of the others mentioned, were obviously quite unusual and therefore no example for ordinary folk. The world cannot, however, be so neatly divided between exceptional people and ordinary people. Abram's wealth did not make it easier for him to move from Haran to Canaan. That move would no doubt have been far easier with fewer sheep, goats and children. Nothing in Sarah's life up to that point fitted her to become a mother at 99. Neither Moses' early life in Pharoah's court nor the years as a shepherd in Midian provided the skills needed to free an enslaved people. Forty years as a chief of landless shepherds in the Sinai wilderness afforded Joshua little preparation for invading Canaan.

It is not important for us to know whether or not these were extraordinary people, or whether they did extraordinary things. What matters is that they were open to God's call, and that they trusted God to provide what they lacked. Our call in later life may not resemble any of theirs in any way except that it comes from God. Our response need not resemble theirs in any way except that we trust God to provide whatever we lack for the task at hand.

NOTES

1. The non-canonical BOOK OF JUBILEES derives its name from the provisions of Leviticus 25:1-17. Every seventh year was to be a Sabbath Year during which the land was to rest as God had rested on the seventh day. Following seven periods of seven years, or seven "sabbaths" of years, there was to be a year of restoration, a Year of Jubilee. The term "jubilee" thus refers to a period of fifty years.

2. The Hebrew word here and elsewhere (e.g., Ruth 3:7 and Isaiah 6:2) trans-

lated "feet" is thought to be a frequent Old Testament euphemism for the sexual organs. Thus, this verse probably indicates that Asa was impotent in old age. *Cf.* O. J. Babb, "Sex, Sexual Behavior" in THE INTERPRETER'S DICTIONARY OF THE BIBLE (New York: Abingdon Press, 1962), IV:298.

3. Of the spies Moses sent into the land, only Joshua and Caleb believed the land could be taken. Only they were spared the penalty that no one then more than 20 years old would enter the promised land (Numbers 14:30). Caleb was then forty years old (Joshua 14:7). Joshua was probably about the same age, since those chosen as spies were already leaders in their tribes (Numbers 13:2). Both remained in the wilderness forty years until Moses and the others had died.

4. Max Weber, THE THEORY OF SOCIAL AND ECONOMIC ORGANIZATION (New York: Oxford University Press, 1947). See also Robert C. Tucker, "The Theory of Charasmatic Leadership" in DAEDALUS, volume 97, number 3, Summer 1968.

Chapter 4

The Play's the Thing

All the world's a stage,
And all the men and women merely players.
They have their exits and their entrances,
And one man in his time plays many parts,
His acts being seven ages.

—Shakespeare, *As You Like It*

We need a framework within which to understand the progress of our growing up. Jacques' melancholy description of the seven ages of man in Shakespeare's *As You Like It* offers a useful insight. Human life is indeed like a play upon the stage. We move through the sixty, seventy, eighty or more years between birth and death as a series of eras or epochs that resemble the acts in a play. The boundaries between the acts are marked by transitions akin to changes in the scenery against which a play is acted. Major historical events alter the shape of our lives as do events that occur offstage or before a play begins.

No two real-life plays are ever quite alike. The roles we play are shaped by the settings in which they are lived out, by others who play key roles, and by the events that become significant moments (*kairoi*). The action within each act is called forth by a unique combination of time and place, heredity and environment. The scenes within which we act out our lives change over the years. There is much, nonetheless, that is similar about all the real-life plays that humans act out.

Men and women are seldom merely players. Few lives resemble a comic opera, fewer still a classic tragedy, yet playwrights draw their raw materials from the stuff of human lives. No real-life play is ever without both crisis and pain. None is lacking in moments of humor and comic relief. However ordinary, there is in every life struggle with the forces of good and evil. There is joy, there is sorrow. There is good fortune, there is ill. There is laughter, there is weeping. Some lives end too soon, before their creative potential is fully realized. Others drag on long after energy and enjoyment are used up. Our lives know birth and death, creation and destruction, hope and despair, longing and regret, love and hate.

That life consists of a series of acts or stages, and that each has its particular themes, is not a new idea. In 44 BC, Cicero wrote: "Every stage of life has its own characteristics: boys are feeble, youths in their prime are aggressive, middle-aged men are dignified, old people are mature. Each one of these qualities is ordained by nature for harvesting in due season."[1] In *As You Like It*, Shakespeare listed seven ages and described them in biting satire: the infant, the school-boy, the lover, the soldier, the justice, the old man, the dying person.[2]

More recently, Erik Erikson described eight stages: infancy, early childhood, play age, school age, adolescence, young adult, adulthood, mature age.[3] Levinson,[4] Sheehy,[5] and others have contributed to a growing body of literature about the stages of human life. For the most part, only the patterns of male life have been studied. Little has been written about the stages of women's lives.[6] While many books have been written about the stages of adult life, little attention has been paid the years beyond retirement.

These discussions of human development are largely descriptive. Any attempts to define normative experience are grounded in empirical observation. Life is usually perceived as a series of stages, with movement from one stage to the next more or less inevitable. Sometimes the individual is seen as having relatively little control over his or her life. There is no significant agreement about how many stages there are or about how movement occurs from one stage to the next.

Life can be described as like a play consisting of several acts and scenes within acts. The roles we are called to play are much the same from one real-life play to the next. There is room for considerable individuality and inventiveness about which roles we choose to play and how we play them. Because the other characters with whom we share life's stage enjoy this same freedom, a good deal of improvisation is necessary. As a result, life can be rich and exciting, filled with surprises and challenges.

TWO NEW ACTS

Until the 20th century most lives seem to have consisted of no more than three acts: childhood, adulthood, and old age. Life usually looked something like this:

Birth	Puberty		Frailty	Death
¦ Childhood ¦		Adulthood	¦ Old Age ¦	

Childhood was often short, and only the children of the well-off got much education beyond the basics of reading, writing and arithmetic. As soon as they were big enough, children often were sent off to labor in their father's or the landlord's fields, or in the nearby mill or factory. Childhood ended with puberty, when boys were deemed old enough to assume a man's responsibilities and girls were considered fit for marriage and childbearing. Though poets sometimes praised its innocence, childhood's chief importance appears to have been preparation for adult life. Children seem at times to have been considered small adults. Medieval artists sometimes painted them that way.

The adult years were often marked by hard physical labor for both men and women. Until the latter part of the nineteenth century, most men were employed on farms or in mills and factories. Animals or machines provided some of the energy, but work was hard and dangerous, and injuries were frequent. Farm women worked alongside their husbands in the fields, or raised gardens and chickens while the men raised field crops and larger livestock. Town women often worked in mills and factories, and their work was also hard and dangerous. Women who worked only at home kept house without today's appliances. Clothes were washed by hand, hung out to dry winter and summer, and made presentable with "sad-irons" heated on the kitchen range. Wood for the range and the parlor stove was chopped by hand, and coal was carried up from a bin in the cellar. Few rural houses had central heat, and none had air-conditioning.

Old age began when the body could no longer sustain the demands of hard work, or when a final illness set in. It was often short, consisting of a period of physical frailty or chronic illness. Retirement existed only for the well-off, although workers injured on the job were sometimes pensioned off. Here and there, as today, some older people remained active until quite advanced ages. Some made notable contributions very late in life to their chosen fields or to civic affairs. For the most part, however, old age had little to commend it. That was not a problem for very many, however, because disease, injury, childbirth, and hard physical labor often ended lives well before the third act.

Within the last hundred years or so, at least two new acts have been added to the typical play. One has developed between the first and second acts, and is commonly called adolescence. The other takes place before the final act. While there is not widespread agreement about what it should be called, in this book it will be referred to as maturity. Now life looks more like this:

Birth	Puberty	End of Schooling	Empty Nest	Retire- ment	Frailty	Death
Childhood	Adolescence	Adulthood		Maturity	Infirmity	

In a sense, adolescence has been around for a long time. The youths often mentioned in ancient Greek literature seem to have been no longer children and not yet adults. Their days were spent developing minds and bodies for adult life. Not until the twentieth century has such a period been a normal part of most American lives, however. Often equated with the teen years, it is probably more accurate to say that adolescence begins with puberty and ends when formal education ceases to be the individual's principal occupation. Its length thus varies considerably.

Adolescence represents a lengthening of the time spent in preparation for adulthood. That this stage has become common in most American lives should probably be attributed to the spread of compulsory education through secondary school, and the increased necessity of college and graduate school as preparation for careers in a highly technological society. Assuming an adult role in today's society requires far more training than was needed to pick up the reins of a farm team or go off to war or to sea as adolescent boys once did; far more than was needed to keep house and bear children as teenage girls once did. The years needed for formal education have therefore grown longer.

In some ways, adolescence represents a lengthening of childhood. Preparation for adult life is seldom completed by puberty. Much of childhood is now spent preparing for more advanced schooling, while higher education is seen as the most important preparation for adult life. Adolescents are not children, however. Puberty marks the end of childhood only because it is the beginning of reproductive capability, an adult function. Adolescents are not fully adults. Most have not taken up the classic forms of adult behavior and responsibility: a fulltime career or trade, and the establishment of a household. Marriage and the bearing of children (once clear marks of adult status) are still important but no longer deemed essential. In today's society they are now deferred until later by some and foregone by others who are in other respects clearly adults.

Adolescence can be understood as a transitional stage, enabling the individual to change from child to adult over an extended period of time. Some spend relatively little time in this period. Leaving school as soon as possible, they assume adult responsibilities not long after puberty. Others spend more than a dozen years in this life stage. Continuing their education at the graduate level, they do not take up typical adult responsibilities until the late twenties. Some mix adolescence and early adulthood, marrying and raising children while still in school. Some leave school but take up none of the characteristics of adult life until years later, remaining, as it were, in continuing adolescence.

Because of its length, it is probably more appropriate to regard adolescence as a full-fledged life period in its own right. Having become the norm for most Americans, adolescence has taken on characteristics markedly different from either childhood or adulthood. Young adolescents sometimes make good use of their similarity to children, while older teens often insist upon being treated as adults. Both are, however, in a life period quite different from other stages.

As adolescence has become more commonly part of our life, social institutions have been created or modified in response to the needs of young people. Dwellings now include a family room separate from the living room, allowing adults and adolescents to pursue their separate interests with lessened conflict. The recording and clothing industries now aim many of their products at a young market. Professions such as psychology and social work include specializations devoted to study and treatment of adolescent problems.

Similar changes have occurred within the church. Youth ministry has become an established program in most congregations, as well as a recognized specialty in parish ministry. Special curriculum materials are produced for youth church school classes and fellowship programs. Summer camping and conference programs are considered an essential adjunct to the congregation's program of youth ministry.

Maturity also has been around for a long time. From ancient times there have always been those who lived far longer than most. While some continued to rear children at advanced ages, most of those who lived longer than others seem to have been no longer actively parents and not yet victim to the frailties and feebleness of old age. Many spent their latter days as tribal leaders, seers and sages, poets and prophets. Not until the 20th century has such a period been a normal part of most American lives, however. There are no clear age boundaries, but it is probably accurate to say that *maturity* begins with the arrival of the *empty nest* and grandparenthood, and reaches fullness with formal retirement. It ends with the onset of final illness, feebleness or frailty.

A lengthy period of maturity has now become common in the United States and in most western nations. This can be attributed to several factors. Few die of childhood diseases today and fewer still carry into adult life their crippling after effects. No longer is it common for one or both parents to die before the last of the children has grown to adulthood. The diseases of the middle years have been brought under better management. Few die of the first heart attack or stroke. New methods of treatment enable many to lead active, productive lives despite diabetes, cancer, and other serious chronic conditions.

It is difficult, if not impossible, to say when maturity begins or ends. Parents of one or two children may experience the empty nest as early as the mid-40s. Retirement most often occurs in the mid-60s. Infirmity often does not begin until the mid-80s. The years of maturity can thus be as many as 40 or more, and are seldom fewer than 20.

Maturity represents more than a lengthening of the adult years, however. Life neither ends nor loses its purpose when the last child leaves home, or when office, store or factory no longer demands five or six of every seven days. Mature people differ from younger adults, however. Those finished with child rearing no longer maintain a household organized primarily for that purpose. Those who have retired no longer pursue a fulltime career or trade. Some, widowed and living alone, maintain a household only in the narrowest sense.

Mature adults often devote far less time than do younger adults to the classic forms of adult behavior mentioned earlier. Finished with child rearing, and no longer required to work, many turn their attention to other concerns. Some turn a large part of their time to new or postponed interests, while others spend much of their time caring for an aging relative. Still others pursue leisure on a fulltime basis. They travel often, or visit their children in serial fashion. For them, home may be only a place to store out of season clothing and pick up the mail from time to time.

Some still think of early maturity, the years just after the last child is grown or the first grandchild arrives, as the beginning of old age and infirmity. Grandparents seldom live "over the river and through the trees" any longer, but are often thought to be slowing down a bit. Gray hair is no sure indicator of either age or incompetence, yet employers think twice about hiring or promoting those with it.

Mature people differ markedly, however, from the very old and infirm. Chronic conditions may call for eyeglasses, regular medications, or occasional therapy, but seldom restrict daily activities. Mature people are neither frail and feeble nor dependent on others. They are occasionally forgetful, as are younger people, but they are not senile. Both Alzheimer's Disease and severe cerebrovascular accidents (strokes), the principal causes of senility, usually occur much later. They affect a rather small proportion of the total age group and are the principal causes of the onset of infirmity.

Later maturity, the years following retirement, is in some respects a transitional stage in which the individual changes gradually from active adult to one who will soon die. Some spend only a short time in this period. Deprived of purpose for their lives by the loss of work through retirement or the loss of their spouse, they find it difficult to recover from a major illness or injury and become frail and dependent. Others take up new pursuits after widowhood or retirement, or increase their involvement in lifelong interests. Some return to school, others take up new careers or become active community volunteers. Remaining in generally good health, they extend their maturity into their 70s, 80s, or even 90s.

Because most people now spend some time in this era between mid-life and infirm old age, it is appropriate to regard maturity as a full-fledged life period in its own right. Having become the norm for most Americans, maturity has begun to take on characteristics which mark it as different from earlier adulthood, as well as from later old age. Mature people often insist upon being treated as middle-aged. Some occasionally find advantage in others' perception of them as old and in need of assistance. In either case, they are in a life period increasingly different from other periods.

As longer life has become more common, social institutions have been modified and others created in response to the needs of those in later maturity. Social security, company and union pensions, various forms of investment, and Medicare, all were developed to provide greater financial security in old age. Nursing homes and retirement homes likewise were developed to care for older people unable to care for themselves. Senior centers, nutrition programs, transportation and escort services, legal assistance and advocacy programs, homemaker and home health services, all have been developed to aid older people needing some help but not requiring institutional care. Commercial products, such as denture adhesives and laxatives, have been developed for an older market. Because the number of older people has grown to unprecedented proportions, some professions now include specializations concerned with study and treatment of the problems of old age.

Attention to the needs and concerns of those in early maturity has developed as well. Retirement housing is now available for those wanting a life style different from those raising families, or those wanting to live in a resort area. Life care facilities offer a comfortable life style and the promise of suitable care when infirmity requires it. Travel opportunities abound and volunteer opportunities have increased markedly. Products like hair coloring and skin cream are popular with those who want to retain the appearance of earlier years. Many professions have paid relatively little attention, however, to the needs and concerns of the active years between adulthood and old age.

The church's response to growing numbers of older people has thus far been mixed. From what began as a few homes built to care for unfortunate and infirm older people, chiefly widows, there has developed a considerable network of retirement and life care homes aimed toward those in later maturity. Denominational social service agencies have initiated relatively few services for mature people. Here and there, camps and conferences for older adults have appeared. Volunteer service programs have made room for increasing numbers of mature volunteers. These programs have been largely outside the local congregation, however, and sometimes have isolated individuals from its life.

Church leaders often reflect society's view of the later years as an unpleasant time to be suffered through. Ministers seldom choose to specialize in older adult ministry. Religious education curricula largely overlook the developmental possibilities in the mature years. Congregational activities usually are planned for families with school age children or for adults in their working years. Few congregations have developed ministries designed to meet the needs and concerns of mature adults. As a result, older adults feel overlooked, misunderstood, and/or unwelcome.

ENTRANCES, EXITS AND INTERMISSIONS

There is a continuous cycle of beginnings and endings within a play. Characters enter and leave the stage, and their presence or absence alters the play's action. Some characters are seen by the audience but not by the players, others are never seen, yet they influence how other actors play their roles. From time to time, the curtain falls or the lights go down to denote the passage of time, or to permit changes in the scenery within which the actors play their roles. During these pauses in the action, the playwright sometimes introduces transitional events which also alter how the characters play their roles. These events are significant in the lives of the characters, but the playwright has chosen to focus on the subsequent development of plot and characters, rather than on the events themselves.

Individuals come and go and events of greater or lesser significance occur throughout our lives. Each encounter, each relationship, each happening changes our lives in some way. Some produce only small adjustments, hardly more than course corrections. We take them in stride with little awareness that life has changed. Other entrances, exits or events radically alter the direction or quality of our lives. They move us into a new era or epoch as surely as raising the curtain or bringing up the lights begins a new act or scene upon the stage. Sometimes disasters and world events rewrite the acts yet to come. Sometimes we encounter people so extraordinary, our lives are never the same.

For the most part, the people whose entrances and exits begin new scenes are ordinary folk. They are parents, children, wives and husbands, grandchildren, teachers and employers. The events which most often mark the major transitions in our lives are likewise ordinary. They are birth, marriage, death, enrolling in school and graduating, beginning a career and retiring from it. The significance of both people and events lies not so much in themselves as in the way they alter the shape and substance of our lives.

Birth raises the curtain on childhood, the first act. The setting is some sort of dwelling. Enter parents and assorted other kinfolk. As the act progresses, the scenery changes to include neighboring houses and shops, a playground, a school, more and more of the surrounding city. The principal characters in this act include grandparents, aunts and uncles, playmates, and authority figures such as teachers, babysitters, bus drivers, and principals. Among the events that bring up the lights on successive scenes are crossing the street alone, the first day at school, summer camp, and discovering the other sex.

At puberty, the curtain rises on the next act, adolescence. The hero or heroine, still a fulltime student, is far from ready for marriage and adult responsibility. Nevertheless, developing secondary sexual characteristics such as female breasts, male facial hair, changes in voice range, thrust the individual into a new epoch. Sexual intimacy is now not only possible, it is fiercely compelling. Some scenes in this act begin with such exciting events as the first big date and the first real kiss. Others begin with more problematic events, the first sexual intercourse, the first pregnancy, the first experimenting with alcohol or illicit drugs. The important characters often include some off-stage heroes, rock musicians, television actors, athletes, and some on-stage potential career models.

As adulthood begins, the major character begins to play multiple roles and has considerable freedom in doing so. The principle parts to be played in act three are spouse, parent, worker. It now becomes more difficult to describe just what brings up the curtain on each successive act. The difficulty stems in part from the reality that one may become both spouse and parent while still otherwise an adolescent. So long as one is still chiefly engaged in formal schooling, or married to one so occupied, full assumption of the adult role has not occurred. On the other hand, one may finish schooling and begin a career thus becoming an adult, without marrying or begetting children.

For this reason, the end of schooling, or rather the beginning of fulltime self-support, seems the most typical curtain raiser for adulthood. Here we become aware of another difference from earlier acts. Even if we consider conception its onset rather than birth, childhood quite clearly begins at a certain time. Puberty normally falls within a short span of time around age 12 or 13. The end of formal schooling and the beginning of work-related fulltime self-support, however, can occur as early as the end of secondary school or as late as the end of post-graduate studies. Adulthood thus often begins as early as age 15 or 16 and as late as age 28 or 29.

At one time, marriage and parenthood (and only in that order) were deemed essential for all adults. There is greater freedom today on both matters. Still, the entrance of a husband or wife, a set of in-laws, and one or more children, is often part of the third act. Whether work, marriage or parenthood raises the curtain, the individual is thrust again into a new era quite different from the one before. There are two principal settings, a dwelling and some sort of workplace. The scenery also includes neighboring houses and stores, playgrounds and schools, and large parts of the surrounding city. Events which bring up the lights on other scenes include job changes, divorce, an accident or a major illness.

The fourth act, which we call maturity, typically consists of two major sub-acts. One, *early maturity*, begins with the end of active parenting, sometimes called the *empty nest* stage. The other, *later maturity*, begins with formal retirement, the end of work-related self-support.

The curtain rises on early maturity when the last child leaves home, establishes a household, marries, or begins fulltime self-support. Our heroine or hero now becomes the parent of adult children. Offspring who have departed the family nest soon produce their own children, and our principal character also becomes a grandparent. With these changes often comes a feeling of release and freedom. Finances are a bit easier now. The scenery may change to include travel or a second home, deferred while the children were finishing their educations. Among the familiar characters in this act are the grandchildren, who can be spoiled with impunity, and who go home at night.

Work usually continues for a few more years. Sometimes both husband and wife are employed. Careers often reach their peak during these years, and individuals sometimes are shunted aside to make room for rising younger colleagues. Among the characters who often appear in this act are the lover or the younger woman. The streaks of gray at the temples and the crow's-feet around the eyes are often accompanied by a crisis of confidence with intimations of one's mortality. Individuals play this scene in a variety of ways.

Since not all adults marry or have children, there are many who do not experience the empty nest or have grandchildren. But siblings, classmates and colleagues do, and nieces and nephews graduate and go to work and marry and have children. Those who never married, and those with no children, have career peaks and crises of confidence. Some have affairs or divorce and remarry; some resume their education or begin new careers. Sometime during these years, most people first become aware that the years yet to come are likely to be fewer than those already lived. The awareness that someday we shall die is a good clue that the curtain has risen on early maturity.

Formal retirement clearly thrusts individuals into a new epoch. In reasonably good health and still able to work, they no longer derive their income from fulltime work. Employers, fellow workers and colleagues, members of the carpool and seatmates on the bus now exit the stage. The husband who left most mornings at 7:30 and returned each evening at 6:00 is now on stage for most of the rest of the act. Parts of the scenery that have been familiar through two acts are withdrawn into the wings. Often, the last scenes of this act must be got through without the husband or wife one has played opposite all these years. Later, maturity includes scenes potentially difficult to play. Nonetheless, many play them with excitement and imagination.

The final act curtain rises to reveal a scene in which the central piece of furniture is often a bed or a wheelchair. Infirmity begins in earnest when physical frailty or severe illness, whether chronic or acute, becomes the dominant factor in the individual's life. Often the hero or heroine must play much of this act alone on stage. The most likely other characters are an aging spouse, a caring daughter or daughter-in-law, home health aides, someone bringing a hot meal, nurses and nurse aides, and doctors. Relatives seen often on stage in earlier acts are sometimes conspicuous by their absence. Sometimes they have died or moved far away. At other times one senses they are in the wings, waiting for their curtain calls, but somehow unable to play this scene. This act can be mercifully short or terribly long. At length, death rings down the final curtain.

AN ANALOGY FOR LIFE

More is written about maturity and infirmity in the chapters which follow. Play and stage are used occasionally as analogies for life and its milieu, but with some reservations. Individual lives seem like plays because art mirrors life. Each life is made up of recognizable periods not unlike the acts in a play, and a succession of acts much the same from one life to the next. People seem "merely players" because the roles that typically fall within certain acts recur, in similar acts, in other real-life plays.

Analogies have limits beyond which prudent writers and readers ought not venture. Life is no situation comedy. There are no stock plots. The roles we play on life's stage are defined by far more than playbooks and rented costumes. Unlike actors, we do not take off our makeup and go home after the final curtain. "Taking off one's makeup and going home" is no fit analogy for resurrection to eternal life, however cute it may be. "Final curtain" falls far short of comprehending the significance of an individual's death. The Old Testament account of Job and his family notwithstanding, God is never so capricious with humans as are the writers of classic tragedies, comic operas, and situation comedies.

The play upon the stage is only an analogy for human life, yet the similarities are powerful. In life, as on the stage, one play seems much like another, yet each is unique, each plot and script partly improvised. In life, as in a well-constructed play, the action builds from the curtain's first rise until it falls for the last time. Each act is different from the others, but each is important to the successful resolution of the plot. Unless playwright and actors create the later acts with as much care as the earlier ones, the play will fail of its purpose.

NOTES

1. "Cato the Elder on Old Age" in Cicero, SELECTED WORKS, translated by Michael Grant (Baltimore: Penguin Books, 1960), 226.

2. Act II, Scene 7, 139-166.

3. Erik H. Erikson, CHILDHOOD AND SOCIETY (New York: W. W. Norton, 1963), 247-274; IDENTITY AND THE LIFE CYCLE (New York: International Universities Press, 1959), 120; INSIGHT AND RESPONSIBILITY (New York, W. W. Norton, 1964), 111-134.

4. Daniel J. Levinson, THE SEASONS OF A MAN'S LIFE (New York: Alfred A. Knopf, 1978).

5. Gail Sheehy, PASSAGES (New York: E. P. Dutton, 1974).

6. However, see Carol Gilligan, IN A DIFFERENT VOICE: PSYCHOLOGICAL THEORY AND WOMEN'S DEVELOPMENT (Cambridge: Harvard University Press, 1982).

Chapter 5

Still Room to Grow

Every transition begins with an ending. . . . First there is an ending, *then* a beginning, with an important empty or fallow time in between.

— William Bridges, *Transitions*

If we marry and set up housekeeping, considerable time and effort are devoted to rearing children during the first twenty or so years of our adult lives. One day the last of our children moves out of the family home and establishes a separate household. The curtain now rises on a new act in our lives, an era marked by adjustments in life style, changes in individual roles, and some degree of disruption and discomfort.

This transition, often called the empty nest, does not begin abruptly, nor is it soon ended. Intimations of its coming are felt as early as the day the last of our children starts to school on a fulltime basis. The fact that changes are occurring becomes more apparent when our youngest child enters adolescence and develops an identity and existence increasingly different from both parents and older siblings. The transition is not complete until the last child establishes a household separate from that of the parents. Even then some unfinished business may remain and may not be resolved for several more years.

Marriage and parenthood are the most frequent choices of adult lifestyle. Many of the midlife changes described in this chapter occur, however, without regard to parenthood. Some of the changes we experience result from changes in health and physical functioning. Those whose energies are heavily invested in vocation or career often experience a severe crisis in the middle years. Many of these changes occur within a relatively short span of years around age 50. Their combined impact upon the individual needs to be considered together with the significance of each particular change.

The experience of the "empty nest" is characteristically accompanied by other changes in the structure and dynamics of marriage and family life, physical capabilities and health, and in the nature and quality of work. These changes bring an awareness that youth has ended. This often provokes a time of individual and interpersonal tumult. All of these events call us to reconsider roles and values adopted earlier in adult life, explore new options and opportunities, and assess our spiritual resources for the journey that lies yet ahead.

CHILDREN BECOME ADULTS

One of the most demanding roles in adult life is entrusted to individuals with no experience. Just when we have become proficient our services are no longer needed. Just when we have finally gotten the hang of being parents, our children become adults. They cease to need or want the close supervision and guidance we have been accustomed to give them. Twenty to thirty years' worth of experience and commitment become unwelcome and useless.

That is how it is when humans reach their late teens and early twenties. An important part of growing up is establishing our own identity apart from our parents. Puberty marks the beginning of a period of getting ready for adult roles and responsibilities. In the years that follow, the forming of an adult identity is a primary developmental task. In part, we accomplish that by setting ourselves over against the adults who have nurtured and cared for us through childhood. By testing their values and their authority we begin to form an identity of our own to which we can be faithful in the years ahead.

The process of becoming an adult is something like a bird's experience of learning to fly. Whether we leap from the nest of our own will or are pushed out by one or both parents, we have to try our wings and discover for ourselves that they will support us, and that we can fly without help. Humans learn more slowly than birds. Our takeoffs and landings are clumsy for quite a while and we run into walls and trees a lot. But the experience is essential. Until we have come to an identity of our own, we cannot exist apart from our parents, we cannot form meaningful alliances with significant others.

Parents often do not accept easily their children's entry into adulthood. Over the years since we began that transition, we have discovered that being an adult is much harder than we first believed. Conscious of our own errors of judgment and missed opportunities, we want to steer our young away from the pitfalls and stumbling blocks we see in their path. Only with difficulty do we step back and allow our children room to make their own mistakes, and learn to be adults on their own.

As children become adults, they begin to use the sexual capability that arrived with puberty. "Thus, the young adult, emerging from the search for and the insistence on identity, is eager and willing to fuse his identity with that of others."[1] Sometimes this part of our children's maturing is the hardest for parents to handle. Through our own adult years we have learned how powerful sexual attraction can be. We bear the scars that show how easily wrong choices are made. Only with difficulty do we keep silent and allow our children to seek the intimacy that is the logical next step in their development.

With maturity comes the need for one's own nest. That too is sometimes hard for parents to accept. The two foot high Christmas tree on your daughter's first coffee table, decked out with a single string of lights and one box of shiny balls, seems pitiful compared to your own eight foot tree which is adorned with a quarter century's accumulated family treasures. Your son's two-room flat, warmed only a little by a space heater, and furnished with a card table, two battered old chairs and a mattress on the floor, seems dreadfully shabby compared to his comfortable room at home.

Only with difficulty do we recall our own salad days, when our worldly treasures consisted of an old trunk, a hope chest, two orange crates and a few boxes of books, and our first home was two bedrooms converted to a small apartment upstairs in an old house. Establishing a household separate from our parents is an important part of becoming an adult. Nonetheless, it is not easy to stand back and watch our children start at the bottom as we once did. We forget how much we valued our independence and how sure we were that we would shortly live more handsomely than our parents.

No matter how much we longed for the time when they would all be gone from the house, the silence can be deafening. We miss the convenience of someone, always eager to drive the family car, to return library books, pick up the dry cleaning, or run to the market for some forgotten item. We miss someone to mow the lawn, trim the hedges, wash the supper dishes or help set the house to rights before guests arrive. We miss the rituals and the needs that gave shape to our daily routine.

When our children were little, "Mommy, look!" or "Daddy, listen!" was a common refrain. As they grew older, their worlds grew larger and they shared less with us. They found new confidants among school friends and after school coworkers. Some of what they kept from us had to do with their developing sexual lives and choices. Sometimes they were silent to spare us hurt or out of respect for values we held that they did not share. As we became aware of this change we knew it was a necessary part of forming their own existence apart from us. Nonetheless, it was sometimes not easy to accept.

As our children become adults we often experience the joy of watching our dreams and hopes take shape. Despite our inexperience, and sometimes without our help, our children turn into adults we are proud to know. They learn from their mistakes, just as we did. They recover from unwise choices and find new directions for their lives, just as we did. Often they surprise us with insights and competence, tenderness and joy, we hardly dared hope for.

Sometimes our children grow into adults we do not like and cannot respect. They adopt life styles that are painful to see, espouse values we abhor, or marry people with whom we feel uncomfortable. Whether their choices are born of rejection for values we prize, or only in response to the world around, our hopes and dreams must be postponed or abandoned. Sometimes no relationship remains possible, and we go our separate ways.

No matter what kind of adults our children become, arrival at the empty nest is always somewhat painful. As they weather each crisis, or fall before it, we cannot avoid wondering whether as parents we were all we might have been. How easily we recall the many times we were unsure of the choices we made or the rules we enforced. Looking back, we ponder whether, if we had done otherwise, a son or daughter might have turned out differently.

Adult children sometimes delay leaving home after formal education has been completed. They avail themselves of their parents' continued support until careers or businesses are well enough established to permit self-support. Some do not leave home until they marry; some stay to care for or provide companionship for a widowed parent.

Some adult children return home when job or marriage fails. When adult children live at home it is seldom on the same terms as when they were children or adolescents. Even when economically or emotionally dependent, adult children usually expect to be recognized as adults who are free to make their own choices and come and go as they wish. Even under these circumstances, parents experience many of the same changes as when children leave home.

CHANGES IN MARRIAGE AND FAMILY

Just as we are struggling to accept the reality that our children have become adults, one of them presents us with our first grandchild. Because popular images equate grandparenthood with being older than we are at the time, this event reminds us that our youth is fast fading away. Nonetheless, most of us approach this new role eagerly. Knowing friends have already assured us that grandparents "have it made" because "the children go home at night!" We look forward with delight to the presence of small children in our lives, without the sometimes awesome responsibilities of parenthood.

Most of us began parenthood using our own parents, and those of our friends, as familiar role models. Many of us take up grandparenthood having known few, if any, of our grandparents. Even if we knew all of them, most of our growing up was most likely accomplished at a geographic or emotional distance from them. On the other hand, if they were a part of our childhood household, their presence may have been accompanied by conflict between them and our parents. In short, most of us become grandparents with less satisfactory role models to emulate than when we became parents.

By the time we become grandparents, our children may have

moved to another state, or even another country, or we may have moved and left them behind. As a result, we may not often see our grandchildren. The expectations, nurtured more by films and books than by our own experience, of milk and cookies, of walks in the woods and visits to museums, of lighthearted moments and serious discussions, may go largely unfulfilled.

If our children divorce, we may find it even more difficult to keep up a close relationship with our grandchildren. The parent with custody may try to break off contact with former in-laws. State laws sometimes provide visitation rights for grandparents as well as for divorced spouses. Such statutes do nothing, however, to overcome the bitterness and hurt that too often accompanies divorce.

Even under the best of circumstances, the arrival of grandchildren alters our relationship with our children. Ideally we expect to share with our children the benefit of our years of experience as parents. To whatever extent they found us wanting as parents, they may resist such input, or even place barriers between us and our grandchildren. On the other hand, they may cast us into a role more suited to retirement, dropping by or leaving the children with us when it isn't convenient, or urging us to visit more often than we can manage.

Increasingly, most of us enter the empty nest years with several of our own and our spouse's parents still living. During these years, however, our familiar and comfortable relationship with them will likely change. Some of the contributing factors are described more fully in Chapters 6 and 7.

Our parents' retirement, especially if buttressed by ample income and even modest savings, may be followed by changes in their life style which we find it difficult to accept. The many possibilities include moving to resort or retirement housing, extensive travel, a return to school or the launching of a new business, taking up volunteer work, or other changes that represent a redirection of life. They also could include withdrawing from community involvements, turning down invitations, losing interest in favorite activities, increasing complaints about health problems, or episodes of depression. In short, our parents' retirement may be accompanied by greater independence or by clear signs of a coming dependence on family members.

During the middle years, both men and women sometimes take on behavior patterns traditionally associated with the other sex. Women become more assertive and less nurturing, while men become more nurturing and less assertive. Probably such changes indicate that traditional behavior patterns are less a matter of gender than of society's expectations and conditioning. Perhaps with maturity we respond less to external pressures and more to our own agendas.

Many couples deliberately change the direction of their lives during the middle years. Wives who laid aside education or career, in response to family needs, often return to school or work. Husbands whose careers require less time and effort than in earlier years sometimes take on added household or community responsibility, especially to support their wives' new ventures.

It should not be supposed that returning to school or work comes easily for women in the empty nest years. Skills and experience acquired many years earlier are likely to be rusty, out-of-date, even obsolete. In some fields, training or formal education once adequate for entry is no longer sufficient for reentry. Work roles and values learned earlier may be out of step in today's world.

Some husbands prefer that their wives remain at home even after the children are grown. A man who views work primarily as a source of income may not understand his wife's desire to find self-fulfillment through work or career. The easing of family finances, as children grow up and complete school, may prompt him to argue that *his* wife doesn't *need* to work. His sense of well-being may be threatened as her earnings lessen her dependence on him.

Most couples begin marriage with the expectation of rearing children. Children usually arrive within a very few years after the wedding. Over the next twenty to thirty years, most couples devote a large measure of their energy and a significant portion of their resources to their children's needs, interests and education. They modify or defer their own wishes and needs until the children are older, or family resources increase.

As the children establish their own households and complete their educations, most parents find they have more time for their own pursuits. If career earnings are also peaking, couples often turn their attention to travel, vacation homes, leisure pursuits, and the like.

After the novelty wears off, some find that without the shared activities and concerns related to childrearing, their marriage lacks the excitement and joy of being together they knew before the children arrived.

Some marriages fail at this point. The stresses of mid-life crisis (see below), changes in individual priorities and values, inattention to the niceties of life together, missed opportunities for affection and intimacy, disputes over personal agendas, the accumulation of slights and hurts, all take their toll.

When marriages end in midlife, it can be without the rancor and bitterness that often surrounds divorce. Some couples simply agree to part because their personal agendas can be pursued more readily apart than together, because they no longer love each other enough, or because there is no longer any compelling reason to remain together. While such divorces appear amiable, and former partners sometimes remain good friends, the separation can be painful, and the transition to new roles and lifestyles can be difficult and confusing.

Midlife marriages are as likely to end in widowhood as in divorce. While life expectancies for both men and women now average more than seventy years, death becomes more common after the late 40s and early 50s, especially among men. The most common causes of death today are heart disease, stroke, cancer, brain disorders such as Alzheimer's and Parkinson's Diseases, and diabetes. Unlike the infectious diseases that were the foremost killers a century ago, these diseases are primarily associated with middle age and later life. Widowhood is more common in the years after retirement, and will be discussed more thoroughly in the next chapter.

Both divorce and widowhood are often followed by remarriage. Men are more likely than women to remarry in the later years. Opportunity is a major factor. Because men generally die earlier than women, the number of widows grows more rapidly from the 50s onward than does the number of widowers. Men, more than women, may also need or prefer marriage. They tend to rely more on the primary relationship with spouse and less on secondary relationships with friends and neighbors than do women. When a man is divorced or widowed, he may therefore feel a greater urgency to replace the lost relationship.

CHANGES IN PHYSICAL STATUS AND HEALTH

Throughout life our bodies undergo change. Rates of respiration and circulation, muscle tone, stamina, ability to handle stress, and a host of other factors, are all affected by life style, diet, environment and disease. During our middle years some more-or-less permanent changes begin to be apparent. Most of these changes do not impose limitations on our ability to function normally at work or at home. Some, especially if not treated or corrected, may in time bring severe limitations.

Changes in vision are often the first to be noticed. The muscles that control the focus of the ocular lens lose some of their strength. Those with relatively normal vision begin to have difficulty reading fine print, especially in dim light. Their difficulty is easily corrected with reading glasses. Those with near-sightedness (*myopia*, literally "closed eyes") find their problem somewhat improved, at least for a time, by the onset of far-sightedness (*presbyopia*, literally "old eyes"). Later, when similar changes in distance vision occur, bifocal lenses provide an effective solution.

Changes in hearing capacity often occur during this time also. Usually the first change to be noticed is some difficulty in discerning what another is saying in a setting where there is considerable ambient noise. Lessened ability to hear certain frequencies of sound makes conversation more difficult at a football game or in a busy restaurant. Initially, these changes cause little difficulty and are dealt with by more careful attention to the other person and some care in choosing the settings for important conversations. Later, a hearing aid may become a necessary, if only partially effective, solution.

These changes in vision and hearing are to be expected and little can be done to prevent them. Changes in muscle tone, physical stamina, circulatory and respiration rates, and general fitness are influenced far more by environment, diet, life style and exercise. As we enter the middle years, our life style is likely to become more sedentary, our diet richer. A middle-age spread and shortness of breath after climbing stairs are good indications that corrective measures are in order. The present popularity of active sports like tennis and swimming, and of jogging, running, and walking, in moderation, contribute to a higher level of general fitness during early maturity.

Chronic conditions become more common during these years and many occur in spite of our efforts to maintain fitness. Elevated blood pressure (hypertension) is the most widespread chronic condition among those in their 50s and early 60s. It can usually be lowered with diet or regular medication, and when controlled usually requires no other changes in life style. Diabetes, small strokes, cancer, and heart disease become somewhat more likely with each advancing year after age 50. If these diseases are detected and treated early, it is often possible to avoid or delay any limitations in work or other daily activities.

Women commonly experience menopause during their late 40s or early 50s. Changes in production of the hormone estrogen during this time often produce severe emotional and physical distress. The loss of childbearing ability is traumatic for some women, signaling as it does an end to one of life's major roles. For others, perhaps most for those with several children, this change marks an end to the fear of unwanted pregnancy, and makes possible new sexual enjoyment and a sense of freedom like that men are thought to enjoy.

About the same time many men experience a decrease in the production of testosterone, with some accompanying loss of sexual potency and performance. These changes do not bring to an end the capacity to beget children but do, nonetheless, lead to a good deal of emotional distress for many men. Perhaps because male sexual performance is short-lived and vulnerable to stress, any decrease in capability is often interpreted as a loss of virility. Fear that such is the case can lead to further loss of function.

These changes clearly signal both men and women that they are no longer young. Implicit in that realization is the belief that one must therefore be old. From every direction come strong messages that it is good to be young, bad to be old. Our speech is filled with stereotypes of old age. To be old is to be worn out, unattractive, incompetent, uninteresting, over the hill, a has-been. In a society that places great value on youth, to come to the end of one's youth can be very traumatic.

MIDLIFE CRISIS

The empty nest has long been seen as a time of crisis for women. When she completes childrearing, a woman loses a major life role. The loss of this function can call into question her status as a woman. In the 1960s, the terms "momism" and "smother love" were applied to women who did not relinquish the parental role. They were seen as manipulative and overbearing. Their behavior toward their adult children, especially their sons, was thought to prevent them from attaining full maturity. They were blamed for their sons' draft evasion or homosexuality, for their daughters' feminism or frigidity.

Until recently society held out few options for women beyond marriage and parenthood. Increased concern for equal treatment of women has opened for many the possibility of lifelong careers. Higher costs for housing, larger expenditures for consumer goods, pressure to send children to college and graduate school, have led many women into the work force. Day care centers have made it possible for women with young children to work fulltime. Others return to work when the children are older. Whether they consider it a career or a necessity, work affords many women an important role alongside parenting, and softens the impact of the "empty nest."

Men often are preoccupied more with their careers than with rearing children. When that is the case, the "empty nest" may make little difference and may pass largely unnoticed. Society does not associate rearing children with being a man. It is assumed therefore that the "empty nest" does not produce in men any significant loss of sexual role. Many men, however, take an active part in rearing and nurturing their children. These men are likely to experience a considerable sense of role loss when the last child leaves home. The frequency with which men experience a midlife crisis focused on sexual potency should lead us to ask whether the end of childrearing could be a factor in the development of that crisis.

The middle years bring increased awareness of the shortness of life. While reading about the latest changes in average life expectancy, or celebrating another birthday, it dawns on us that we have passed life's midpoint. The years that remain are likely to be fewer than those already past. Too few of youth's dreams have come to pass. The greater half of what we set out to do remains unfinished.

The sense of our own mortality is further heightened when co-workers and siblings succumb to life-threatening illnesses. Until this century, death was common at every age. Now it is confined largely to the later years. As a result, apart from wartime, few experience the death of someone their own age until middle age. Even the death of a parent seldom brings home to us the inevitability of our own death as does the death of a colleague or close associate.

Attainment of seniority or advancement to a management position brings increased responsibilities at work, but with it comes the departure of older and more experienced workers to whom we could always turn for advice and support when our experience was inadequate. Once we have taken their place, the expectations of employer and fellow workers can be a source of increased stress. It is not at all unlikely for such a promotion to bring us to a level of lesser competence.[2]

The combination of midlife's many changes can bring a sense of being caught in a no win situation. Changes in family life, lessened physical capacities, the discovery of a chronic health problem, unresolved conflict with a marriage partner, increased responsibilities at work, overlaid with a sense of failure, can stretch to the breaking point one's ability to cope.

Faced with such stresses, many break out in full scale mid-life crisis. Alcohol and drug abuse, extramarital affairs, and playing the market with company funds are but a few of the ways we try to shore up a sagging self-image. Others try instead to start over. Walking out on a failed marriage or a busted career may be easier than setting things to right, but it won't turn the clock back or eliminate the stresses of midlife.

LEARNING TO GROW OLDER

The mid-life crisis is such a popular theme in contemporary fiction that it can become a self-fulfilling prophecy. That is, expecting the normal transitions of mid-life to evoke a personal crisis, we can set ourselves up to respond to them by engaging in dysfunctional behavior.

The transitions of mid-life are real. They include children growing up and leaving home, birth of grandchildren, changes in sexual function, onset of chronic illness, widowhood or divorce, career changes, death of an older mentor, returning to school or to work, and a host of other changes. However, the crises that so readily follow such changes are not inevitable. They tend to grow out of a lack of awareness that a transition is occurring, a lack of interpersonal support, and too little understanding of how to deal with such changes.

When life's transitions occur, we experience in some measure the successive stages—denial, anger, bargaining, depression, and acceptance—of the bereavement process described by Kübler-Ross.[3] The transitions of mid-life have an impact similar to the death of a loved one. After two or three decades our children go away. No matter how vital our relationship with them as adults, as parents of our grandchildren, the children they were are gone, never to return. A marriage of similar duration ends in divorce or death. No matter how amiable the relationship with the former spouse, no matter how much death represents the other's release from pain and suffering, there is loss and there is bereavement.

At such times we focus attention on the ending that is occurring. Our life seems ended, too, and there is little in our experience to tell us otherwise. Day by day, our life goes on. "First there is an ending, *then* a beginning, with an important empty or fallow time in between."[4]

Beginnings seldom come easily, and they can't be hurried. Before we can move forward, we must cease looking backward (Luke 9:62). Before we can relate to our children as adults, we must deal with the end of *their* childhood and *our* role as parents of children. Before we can function effectively as a single adult, or begin a new relationship, we must let go of the now ended marriage and our role as husband or wife. Returning to school may require an end to league bowling or television viewing several evenings each week. Looking for a new job may call for wearing a suit or shaving off a beard worn for a decade. Beginning a new career may mean ending accustomed patterns of keeping house and fixing meals.

Such endings can be unsettling, even frightening. We tend to cling to people, places, clothing, behavior that are familiar and comfortable, that help us know who and where we are. The confusion and disorientation we experience is an important part of growing up. Accepting and working our way through the endings that are part of life's transitions calls for a certain amount of introspection. Such reflection is good when it leads to acceptance of the ending and change that has occurred. It fails when it only leaves us wondering whether the change was worth the trouble, or wishing in vain it could have been avoided.

Transitions — some of great consequence, most relatively minor, all important — occur throughout life. Only with some difficulty do most of us come to understand that how we are affected by a particular transition may bear little relation to the event that triggered it. In that respect, as in so many others, our lives are more like situation comedies than classic tragedies.

When we are young, our transitions are so often marked by eagerness for the beginning that is occurring that we fail to take seriously, or deal with, the endings that are occurring. Bridges describes a woman, unsettled by the demands of her newborn, who had not dealt with the end of her freedom to come and go as she pleases or to enjoy uninterrupted intimacy with her husband.[5]

In later life, our transitions are often characterized by an intense awareness that an ending is occurring, accompanied by the assumption that no beginning is possible.

> The transitions of life's afternoon are more mysterious than those of its morning, and so we have tended to pass them off as the effects of physical aging. But something deeper is going on, something as purposive in its own way as the development of social roles and interpersonal relationships in life's first half. It involves letting go of a particular kind of self-image and style of coping with the world. Seldom done in any single time of transition, this is the developmental business of life's second half.[6]

The transitions of later life are not wanting in potential beginnings. Rather, the scripts for adult life which we have carried around with us since our childhood are missing the pages that follow after the curtain comes down on the scenes that deal with raising children. We are left with no score for the entr'acte, no directions for the changes of scene and costume that must occur before the curtain comes up again on the acts that begin with retirement.

The years from empty nest to retirement can be a time of waiting for the other shoe to fall, or a fallow time marked at one end by a major ending, at the other by a significant new beginning. *If people grow older because God has a purpose for old age* (as I proposed in Chapter 2) *then these years provide opportunity for learning to grow old*. With the children grown and out of the house, with retirement still a few years off, it is time to reconsider life's purpose, time to put closure on some aspects of life, time to ready ourselves for whatever God has in mind for the years that lie ahead.

Rethinking the purpose of life involves reconsidering in particular the life task Erikson calls *generativity*. While primarily a concern for "establishing and guiding the next generation, . . . generativity is meant to include such more popular synonyms as *productivity* and *creativity*. . . ."[7] It arises out of our need to be needed. It finds expression in the ingenuity possible in almost every kind of work or avocation, but takes form most readily in the function and tasks of parenthood.[8] It is in this regard that it occupies a particularly important place in the years that follow marriage and the establishment of a household.

More than almost anything else we do, it is through our children that most of us experience the act of creativity, and the responsibility of caring for what we have created. In time, as we have seen, our children outgrow the need for our hands-on nurture. As they establish their own identity apart from us — as they marry, establish separate households, and bear children of their own — they distance themselves from our care. Their departure from the nest reopens the issue of our generativity.

The creativity and energy that has been directed toward the nurture of our children must now be redirected lest we fall into that "stagnation and personal impoverishment" which for Erikson is the alternative to generativity, and tends to be characterized by self-absorption and self-indulgence.[9] It is appropriate to wonder whether the vacation homes, boats, recreation vehicles, extended travel, and other luxuries often evident during later middle age represent the best resolution to the need to redirect one's generativity. Surely such wondering is legitimated by bumper stickers that read: "I'm spending my children's inheritance."

Rethinking life's purpose also requires reassessing how we meet our fundamental needs for love and esteem.[10] Children afford ample opportunities to love and be loved. As children leave the nest the daily expressions of love and caring leave with them. As they become more involved in their own adult lives, they return for a visit less often, forget our birthdays, no longer share important holidays with us. Such changes are both natural and desirable, but the experience of loving and being loved may get lost.

The family bonds that develop while children are growing up contribute to our sense of belonging. As our children grow, much of the sense of family loyalty that once tied us to our parents may be turned toward our own nuclear family. As children leave the nest, bond themselves to new mates, and beget children of their own, our sense of belonging may grow uncertain. When marriages end and elderly parents die during these years, the sense of no longer belonging anywhere may be quite severe.

Through our children we also meet somewhat our need for esteem. When they excel in school or in competition, in the arts or in business, especially in activities where success once was ours, we experience not only self-esteem but the esteem of others as well. Conversely, when they do poorly, or get in trouble, our sense of esteem suffers. Once they leave the nest, and their success becomes more clearly the result of their own endeavors, and less the consequence of our daily nurture, we lose some of our ability to experience esteem from their endeavors.

As younger adults, establishing families and careers, it was appropriate to invest much of our energy and resources within the relatively small worlds of household and workplace. The task now before us is to find new venues for our generativity, to establish new ways of meeting our needs for love and esteem, beyond the confines of our nuclear family. With retirement, we must move also beyond the confines of our present workplace.

As people of faith, we must now also set about to discover God's unique call — a call specifically for each of us and no other — beyond the parenting and work which until now have occupied much of our time and consumed much of our energy. Because parenting and work are demanding, and because society depends upon both for survival, it is inevitably a call for our old age. Only when we have fulfilled our biological and social obligations as parent and worker, can we preoccupy ourselves with *this* call to the exclusion of others.

How are we to discover this personal call? If it seems that God has not left us enough information, we may need first to upgrade our relationship with God. Too often the demands of work and parenting leave little time for spiritual growth. There is time now for our perception of God to grow beyond that of one who makes and enforces rules, who rescues us when we are in trouble and fixes things when they are broken.

God has, in truth, left us more than enough information. In the pages of holy scripture and the pages of our daily newspaper are more than enough clues to both the nature of God and the unique mission to which each is now called. We are not left to wrestle alone, however, with the question of our future. Through our relationship with the church, through its pastoral nurture and its rites and sacraments, together with our own study and prayer, we can discover God's call for our later years.

NOTES

1. Erik H. Erikson, CHILDHOOD AND SOCIETY (New York: W. W. Norton, 1963), 163.

2. Laurence J. Peter and Raymond Hull, THE PETER PRINCIPLE: WHY THINGS GO WRONG (New York: William Morrow and Company, 1969).

3. Elisabeth Kübler-Ross, ON DEATH AND DYING (New York: MacMillan, 1969), 38-137.

4. William Bridges, TRANSITIONS: MAKING SENSE OF LIFE'S CHANGES (Reading, Massachusetts: Addison-Wesley, 1980), 18.

5. *Ibid.*, 10-11.

6. *Ibid.*, 46-47.

7. Erikson, CHILDHOOD AND SOCIETY, 267.

8. Erik H. Erikson, INSIGHT AND RESPONSIBILITY (New York: W.W. Norton, 1964), 130.

9. *Ibid.*; CHILDHOOD AND SOCIETY, 267.

10. See Abraham H. Maslow, MOTIVATION AND PERSONALITY (Second Edition) (New York: Harper and Row, 1970) 35-51.

Chapter 6

More Growing to Do

The Lord said to Abram, "Leave your native land, your relatives, and your father's home, and go to a country that I am going to show you. . . . When Abram was seventy-five years old, he started out from Haran, as the Lord had told him to do. . . .

—Genesis 12: 1, 4

Unless we are very rich, or very poor, work is a central feature of our adult lives. Nearly all men, and well over half of all women, work for wages during most of their years between ages 18 and 65. While we are still engaged in formal education, work begins to define our existence and the nature of our being. For the next forty to sixty years, it occupies a major portion of our waking hours. One day, sometimes without warning, our relationship to the world of work is severed or truncated by retirement. We now begin, in earnest, that act we have labeled *maturity*.

Retirement is likely to be a more abrupt transition than the emptying of the nest described in the preceding chapter. If we are fortunate and prudent, we will anticipate this day and plan for the changes it will bring. Whether planned for or unexpected, retirement will disrupt our established life style and set us apart from those whose lives are primarily occupied with rearing children and career or vocation.

Some of the transitions described in this chapter are not related directly to retirement, but typically occur around the same time in life, often with similar disruption of the individual's and family's life style and routine. In addition to understanding the potential impact of each transition, we need be cognizant of their combined effect on the quality and direction of our lives.

We are likely to approach retirement with the expectation that at long last we will get to do what we want, apart from the influence and expectations of others that have constrained us since childhood. After fifty or sixty years of mostly doing what others require, however, we will find few guidelines and role models for life in retirement. Without thought and planning, we may be unprepared to make creative use of the years that remain.

One change is certain, however, and it is best that we face it at the outset. From now on, we must now describe ourselves as older adults. From the time our last child establishes a household separate from ours, and certainly by the time we have retired from the work force, older is an adjective aptly applied to distinguish ourselves from our children and from *younger* adults primarily concerned with launching careers and starting families. Over the years, society has attached many stigmas, supported by inappropriate stereotypes, to the terms *old* and *older*. Now that we belong to the generation to which these terms apply, we shall best be rid of the stigmas by owning the labels and giving the lie to the stereotypes.

RETIRING FROM WORK

Except for part-time jobs while we are still in school and entry-level or trainee positions, work is seldom entrusted to those with no experience. Education today is heavily concerned with preparing us to enter the work force. Elementary and secondary schools are intended to ready us for college, college for graduate school, and graduate school for an academic, business or professional career. Unlike the British system, where early examinations stream young people toward trade or craft on the one hand, and business or professional career on the other, the earlier one drops out of formal education in the United States, the less likely one is to ever secure permanent employment.

Once we have completed school and begun our first job in earnest, we spend much of the next forty years or so acquiring and perfecting knowledge and skills in an ever-narrowing part of the world of work. Just as we reach that level of competence which in the medieval craft guilds would have entitled us to the title m... just when we are at the peak of our ability and able to teach it to others, it's time to retire.

Our employer begins pressing us to take advantage of the company's generous early retirement package, and we have an uneasy feeling that if we don't take it, we might be laid off in a few months and lose our retirement benefits. We explore openings with other firms in our field, and are told we are over-qualified. We return to work after a bout of angina, or a heart attack that left little damage, to face suggestions that it may be time to do more fishing. Our mailbox and in-basket begin to be full of folders about tours to exotic places, retirement communities, and life insurance for those aged 50 to 80.

Whatever the scenario, we soon discover that a lot of people are beginning to think of us as over the hill, and our skills and experience as out of date. "Don't trust anyone over 30"[1] has given way to "thirtysomething"[2] and federal law has prohibited age-related discrimination in the work place for more than twenty years.[3] Nonetheless, conventional wisdom and age bias still combine to urge most people toward retirement between age 55, when many early retirement plans first become operative, and age 65, when full Social Security benefits become available.

Leaving one's workplace after forty or so years brings a number of changes which we may not anticipate and for which we may be ill prepared. We can plan for some of these changes by taking part in retirement preparation seminars offered by our employer or through a national or community group concerned with the needs of older adults. If retirement is early or unexpected and in any sense involuntary, there may be no opportunity to plan for it. It is even more important, then, that individuals and their pastors understand the impact of the changes retirement will bring.

Work provides us with a purpose for our days and a sense of identity. In addition, it provides an income and fringe benefits such as insurance and travel. It is a schedule which includes leisure time in the form of coffee breaks, days off, and vacations, a place where we belong, relationships with other people, a place in the pecking order, and a sense of belonging in both the world of work and the larger community.

The sense of purpose related to work can begin in childhood or adolescence and may be rooted in the values we seem to learn when very young. Children often choose the same vocation as an admired parent, sometimes to merit the parent's approval, sometimes to perpetuate the parent's values and ideals. Thus, one may choose to join and hope eventually to take over a parent's business concern, another elect to follow a parent's career in teaching or medicine. Often such choices require long years of preparation during which the initial values and ideals are strongly reinforced through the socialization that often takes place during career-oriented formal education.

When the initial values and ideals are further reinforced over the years by a growing sense of mastery, the sense of purpose associated with one's work can become very strong. When such work comes to an end, even when the ending is anticipated and planned for, and especially when it is neither, there may follow an almost overwhelming sense that life has lost its meaning and direction. Professionals thus often seem to have more difficulty retiring than do blue- or pink-collar workers, and often never completely retire but continue to consult or practice on a reduced scale.

The loss of purpose, meaning and direction associated with retirement can be devastating. The high value American men tend to place on success achieved through assertion and competition may add to the likelihood of a sense of great loss after retirement. The high frequency of suicide among older men[4] may be associated in particular with the loss of purpose, meaning and direction after retirement. Preparation for retirement, and any counseling afterward, should address issues of purpose and meaning as well as financial planning.

Formation of a sense of identity in relation to our work begins early and follows a pattern similar to the development of the self-understanding which enables us to be effective as parents. In the latter instance, puberty completes our sexual development as either male or female. Owning that identity enables us to establish intimacy with another of the opposite sex. That leads to the birth of children, and through the rearing of offspring we develop the capacity to nurture what we have produced.[5]

With respect to work, the process begins with "the establishment of a good initial relationship to the world of skills and tools, . . . "[6] The capacity for fidelity, so important to the intimacy of marriage and the responsibilities of parenthood,[7] makes possible the commitment to craft, trade or vocation that leads to mastery and to "man's *love for his works and ideas* . . . , and the necessary self-verification which adult man's ego receives . . . from his labor's challenge."[8]

Family, religion, place of origin, ethnic heritage, accomplishments in athletics or military service, and election to public office can all form the basis of one's identity. Most Americans, however, seem to derive their strongest sense of identity from the work they do. The ending of that work is often similar in emotional stress to the death of a loved one. The new retiree usually experiences in some degree all the stages of loss described by Kübler-Ross: denial and isolation, anger, bargaining, depression, and finally acceptance.[9] When death takes away a loved one or dear friend, the mourner may get stuck in one of these stages. If the sense of identity related to work or career is very strong, the new retiree may need help to work through to acceptance, so that life can go on.

A fortunate few derive most of their income from inheritance or investments. A somewhat larger group depend mostly on Aid to Families with Dependent Children, more commonly known as Welfare. Most of us secure our living from our own or our spouse's work. When we retire that income stops. For all except those whose engagement in work has been limited and sporadic, wages are replaced by Social Security benefits. For some, chiefly those employed over longer periods by larger corporations, wages are also replaced by a private pension. Those not entitled to Social Security benefits often receive Supplemental Security Income, once known as Aid to the Aged, Blind and Disabled.

Some older people, chiefly those with income from investments and private pension, enjoy a comfortable or affluent life style in retirement but this is only for a small percentage of older adults. Most get by on less income than before retirement, yet its purchasing power grows ever smaller as they grow older. Expenses associated with going to work are eliminated, and income taxes are usually lower, but out-of-pocket expenditures for medical care not covered by Medicare rise with age. Income after retirement averages forty per cent less than prior to retirement. Social security benefits barely prevent poverty, and are the sole source of income for a sixth, the primary source for a third, of the elderly. Private pensions provide only a small share of older people's income, and only one in four receive any income from such sources.[10]

Fringe benefits, such as group health insurance, magazine subscriptions, membership in trade or professional associations, and work-related travel, usually end with retirement. Reduced income and benefits, especially when coupled with rising outlays for health care, usually mean fewer options for fully enjoying one's retirement years.

The schedule and pace of our work — Monday through Friday, nine to five, or some similar schedule — provides a circadian rhythm for our lives. When we retire the absence of that rhythm can add stress where none seems warranted, disturb established household routines, and disrupt interpersonal relationships. Under the work ethic, coffee breaks, days off and vacations have become a kind of legitimate leisure warranted because it makes workers more efficient and keeps the industrial machine running smoothly. In retirement, leisure may lose its validity. After a few months we may ask, "What do you do with yourself when every day is Saturday?"

Work also affords us a place to go to, a place where we belong, away from home. Work provides status, a place where we belong in society and in its pecking order. Work often involves a formal or informal code of ethics that defines appropriate behavior. Retirement strips these away, and can lead to feelings of rootlessness, rolelessness, and anomie.

Work establishes a set of interpersonal relationships with co-workers, clients or customers, fellow commuters, people we see every day at the news stand, the lunch counter and all the other places we frequent in connection with our daily routine. We become involved in their lives and they in ours. When we retire, we stop seeing most of them. To make up for their absence, we may overload the few relationships that remain, particularly those within the nuclear family.

BUT NOT FOR LUNCH!

Retirement affects spouses as well as workers. Employed spouses with their own careers are affected as much as full-time home-makers though the particular effects may differ.

A spouse whose place in the community social order is based on the worker's place of employment or position may find that place gone or altered following retirement. A spouse accustomed to an active social life among the worker's colleagues and their spouses may find that life curtailed once retirement has occurred. Or the quality of interaction may be altered once the worker is no longer privy to the daily changes in office or warehouse politics.

The reduction in income that usually follows retirement can also alter the spouse's life style. Opportunities to accompany the worker on work-related travel will be gone. So too will be gatherings with fellow spouses at annual conventions or trade association meetings. Spending for clothing, entertainment and trips to visit the grandchil-dren may all have to be reduced. As expenditures for health care rise later in retirement, still other options may have to be curtailed. In short, the spouse's life space and style may be reduced as much as the worker's.

If the spouse is younger, and not yet entitled to draw Social Secu-rity or pension benefits along with the retiree, it may be necessary for the spouse to return to work to augment a more limited retire-ment income until the spouse also reaches retirement age. The need to rely on the spouse's income to eke out inadequate retirement benefits can exacerbate feelings of loss of identity and purpose al-ready at work in retired person. At home alone all day, lacking the order and activity work once provided, the former worker may turn to alcohol or drugs to ease feelings of inadequacy and uselessness.

A wife's routine is often keyed to her husband's. The hours when he is at work afford time for her career or concerns. Once the chil-dren are gone greater investment of time and energy may enable her career to blossom. Or she may devote greater time to community activities or volunteer service. A husband who is home all day and has yet to find involvements of his own that replace those once associated with his work, may resent or resist his wife's activities.

He may insist that she retire, too, and join in his retirement activities. He may expect her to run errands and carry out his wishes as his secretary or assistant once did. He may even intrude on her private domain of housekeeping, social activity, or community service, offering to organize it for her. More than one wife, confronted with this prospect, has been heard to complain, "I married him for better or for worse, but not for lunch!"

WIDOWHOOD

Next to retirement, widowhood is the most common transition of later maturity, and it affects women far more often than men. Half the women over age 65, two thirds of those over age 75, are widowed. By contrast, only 13.7 percent of the men over age 65, 22.5 percent of those over age 75, are widowed. Three fourths of the men over age 65, two thirds of those over age 75, are married and living with their spouses.[11]

Three factors account for most of these differences. First, men commonly marry women some years younger than themselves. In first marriages, the difference is about three years. In second marriages the difference is often much greater. Second, women live longer than men. Currently, women can expect to live an average of seven years longer than men. Life expectancy for both men and women is likely to increase over the coming decades, though not as rapidly as earlier in this century, and the age gap is expected to widen to eight years.[12] Add the difference in age to the greater longevity, and women can expect to outlive their husbands at least ten years. Third, men are more likely than women to remarry after the death of a spouse or a later life divorce. Men seem to find it less acceptable to live alone than do women. It is socially more acceptable for an older man to marry a much younger woman than for an older woman to do the same. As men grow older, the difference in longevity causes the number of unmarried younger women to grow steadily larger. It is also more acceptable for a man rather than a woman to propose marriage. As a result, men usually find it easier to remarry later in life than do women.

Few, if any, desire widowhood and fewer still seem to prepare for it, even though its likelihood should be readily apparent to most women of middle and later years. Perhaps the reluctance to anticipate and plan for widowhood results from an unwillingness to consider the death of one's mate. We marry by choice, and marriage, even at its worst, is laden with positive and powerful associations. Our partner is someone to whom we were passionately attracted at the outset, and whom we have learned to love more deeply over the years. Together we have shared a home and brought children into the world. We have watched them grow up, marry and repeat the cycle. It can never be easy to contemplate life apart from one we love and with whom we have shared so much.

Some, more often during the empty nest years than later, are widowed abruptly. When an individual dies suddenly in the late fifties or early sixties, it is most often because of a massive heart attack and there has likely been no clear indication that this should be expected. There is therefore no opportunity for the survivor to anticipate the loss, and no particular reason to plan for it in a day when most can expect to live well into their seventies and eighties. Often, when such a death occurs, the couple have been anticipating and planning for the retirement years they expect to spend together. The loss of life partner is thus accompanied by the loss of that future. While relatively few lose their spouses with no warning,[13] those who do must deal with the lack of forewarning and the absence of any preparation.

At the other extreme are those situations in which the death of the spouse is expected and brings to an end a struggle with health problems that has altered each partner's life style as well as their relationship. Nearly half of all situations fit this pattern, and "death is the final release from the pain and suffering experienced by the deceased as well as the survivor."[14] Where the illness attacks the brain, as is the case with Alzheimer's Disease, the survivor may have had to adjust to the partner's loss of memory, recognition, and the ability to communicate. Where the disease destroys the body, as with cancer, there may be great relief that the loved one's severe pain is now ended.

In any event, illness will likely have been the dominant theme in the couple's relationship over a number of years. It will have interfered with daily activities, and required changes in long range plans for enjoying retirement together. Care will have been provided at home for months or years. Toward the end, nursing home care may have become necessary and its financial burden caused further unwanted adjustments in life style. Medicare does not usually pay for the cost of such care, and medical assistance benefits (Medicaid) may not be available without the near impoverishment of the healthy spouse.

When death finally comes, adjustment may be more difficult than when there is no warning. With the latter, feelings of loss center primarily around absence of the loved one, failure to clear up any misunderstandings or declare one's love, and the end of the role of spouse. Where there has been long illness, the new widow or widower must also cope with the reality that life has been organized for some time around a caregiving role now no longer needed, and may be left with finances so depleted that there can be little hope for the future.

In other experience, also nearly half of all situations,[15] illness precedes death, but the death is unexpected. Either the illness is not perceived as life threatening, or the severity of the health condition is unknown to the couple. Chronic problems such as high blood pressure, heart disease, and diabetes can be under control for years, then unexpectedly worsen. Others, such as cancer, can spread suddenly to vital organs without visible symptoms so that death comes without warning.

In such cases, the couple's life style may have been modified somewhat to compensate for the chronic problem, but life was not reorganized around the caregiving routine. Plans for the future may have been limited because of the disease but death was not expected soon and the partners looked toward a future together. Adjustment here is like that when death is sudden, but may include regrets and guilt associated with a belief that death could have been averted if more attention had been paid to the illness.

Learning to be a widow or widower usually follows the stages associated with dying and death described by Kübler-Ross: denial and isolation, anger, bargaining, depression, and acceptance.[16] In addition to mourning a great loss, we must learn to go on living in a life style not of our choosing. Individuals cope with this need in a variety of ways. Some remarry, others would remarry but cannot find a partner, still others settle into a single life style that works for them.

Those who remarry, and those who would like to, must do something with their memories of the former spouse. Marriage is such an intimate and intense relationship that its accumulation of memories, both pleasant and unpleasant, are not easily cast aside. The good times and the bad have become a part of who we are and we can scarcely describe ourselves to someone new without telling our favorite anecdotes about the past. But told too often or with too little sensitivity, such tales may turn the former spouse into an unwelcome intruder in any new relationship.

Sometimes the survivor, sometimes the children, so idealize their memories of the dead spouse or parent, that remarriage becomes impossible. Prospective partners fall short of the standards we hold up beside them. Children demand to know, "How can you do this to Dad? to Mom?" Rather than cross them, rather than risk losing their love, we settle for less than the bright new future we had hoped for. Or we stop half-way to the altar because we can't bring ourselves to replace the lost loved one, no matter how attractive and desirable the prospective partner may appear.

Widows must also adjust to many of the changes associated with retirement described earlier in this chapter. Social security benefits can drop sharply, and income from a private pension stop completely, if benefits were not arranged for the worker's survivor. Widows may find it difficult to maintain once close relationships with their husbands' former colleagues and their wives. An attractive widow may become an unwelcome extra at social gatherings with couples that once were close friends.

Adjustment to widowhood is also difficult because it requires time. Marriage is not only intimate and intense, but often long-lasting. The home where once we heard the other's voice, sensed the other's presence, is silent now, yet filled with shared memories and shared possessions. At first, time and space are filled with those who share our loss and want to ease its pain. Family members and neighbors gather, bringing food, to reminisce. Their support tends to dwindle away, however, long before our need for it is ended.

Women seem to fare better than men at this point. Many a man has a strong, supportive relationship only with his wife. When she is gone, there is no one to whom he can turn. He has forgotten how to form new relationships and doesn't want to be a burden to one he scarcely knows. Women more often have close relationships with other women, especially daughters and daughters-in-law, and turn to these women for the support they need. Nonetheless, both women and men can benefit from groups in which widowers/widows support each other while all learn to cope with their new situation.[17]

CARING FOR ELDERLY PARENTS

Caring for aging parents is another common experience of the retirement years. Many couples arrive at their own retirement with one or more living parents. It is likely that at least one of the surviving parents will be dependent on others for some of their daily needs. Nearly half of all individuals over age 85 are unable to perform one or more personal care activities without help, and more than half are unable to carry out one or more home management activities without assistance. Fewer than a fourth of those over age 85 are patients in nursing homes; others needing help must be cared for at home.[18]

Caregiving is largely a family matter. As many disabled older people are cared for by families at home, as are cared for in nursing homes. If all assistance with personal and household activities is taken into account, families care for three times as many older people as do nursing homes. Most older men are married and live with their wives, while most older women are widowed and live alone. Older men are most likely to receive needed care from their wives; older women most often turn to daughters and daughters-in-law.

As a result, the majority of caregivers are women, and most live with the person they care for. Care is provided seven days a week. Time spent in caregiving averages 12 hours weekly, and increases as the recipient grows older. Two-thirds of all family caregivers are married, and more than half have children under age 17 in the household. Half are employed, but nearly three-fourths report time lost from work because of caregiving. Nearly two-thirds incur additional expenses averaging more than one hundred dollars per month.[19]

The demands of family caregiving can drain family financial resources, exhaust reserves of physical and emotional energy, and cause plans for enjoying retirement to be postponed or scrapped. Families often take into their home a parent needing care hoping to save time and money. Time used for caregiving is thus spread throughout the day and night and may come to be resented more by the caregiver's spouse and children. The parent's needs may require the caregiver to take time off from work, and eventually lose the job or decide to quit. Family income is thus affected by the loss of earnings as well as the actual expenses of care. This too may be resented by family members when entertainment is foregone and needed purchases must be postponed.

The caregiver engages in a juggling act as she tries to meet the needs of both the dependent parent and other family members. Caring for an aging parent was not part of her plans for these years and she may resent the time and money spent on that care. If the one receiving care is her parent, she may feel resentment, even anger, because the one to whom she has always turned to for care and support now requires the same of her and is no longer able to respond to her needs. The anger she feels, while understandable, can thus contribute to further feelings of guilt, because, after all, it isn't Mother or Dad's fault that they need help. If the one cared for is her husband's parent, she may also feel resentment toward her spouse to whatever extent she perceives that he is failing to share the burden.

Caregiving can also be awkward. Older people sometimes need, and resent or are embarrassed about needing, care like that given to an infant. They have not entered a second childhood, however, but are adults whose ability to care for themselves is limited by disease or frailty. The care we provide may resemble how parents care for children, and may even include assuming some financial or legal responsibility for them, but we do not become their parents. They remain our parents, and there is no role reversal. When parents resist our care or complain about decisions we made in good faith and out of concern for their well-being, we are likely to feel anger.

If we display that anger, and they respond with hurt or confusion, we are likely to feel guilt over our anger. The guilt and anger can become a cycle that feeds on itself and snowballs out of control.

Few people like nursing homes, and fewer still want to live in one or place a parent there. The popular perception that families casually dump their elderly into nursing homes is far from the truth. Most families put off such a decision until long after it should be considered. Often institutional care is put off until after care needed exceeds their ability to provide, the cost of care depletes the family's savings, the parent's needs exhaust the caregiver's emotional and physical resources, and usually the caregiver has gone far beyond what s/he can reasonably manage.

Family caregivers and other family members need support with their caregiving, occasional respite from its burden, help coping with their anger and guilt, assistance with care that is beyond their ability, someplace to borrow things like hospital beds and walkers, and information and support when facing major decisions such as selection of a nursing home.

CHANGES AND ADJUSTMENTS

Maturity, the life stage that begins with the departure of the last child from the family nest, and takes shape in earnest when we retire, necessitates a number of transitions that are sometimes difficult and complex. They can be emotionally devastating. Most of us need information, advice and support as we work our way through these changes and adjustments.

The transitions of our earlier years are often equally complex and difficult. They are on the ascendant side of our image of life as a bell-shaped curve. They require that we take on new roles, learn new skills, expand our horizons. They contain all the signs of growing up that we began to anticipate when still very young. The elements of marriage and family on the one hand, work and career on the other, combined with faith in ourselves and in the social and economic systems we are a part of, form an overall dynamic of hope.

As our children graduate from school, distinguish themselves in athletic or academic undertakings, secure employment and launch their own households and families, and as our own careers reach higher levels of success and economic reward, we seem to arrive at the peak of the mythical bell-shaped curve. "It doesn't get any better than this!" may be our slogan as we begin the changes associated with maturity. These transitions seem to belong to the descending side of the curve, and are characterized solely by loss of role and function, decline of knowledge and skills, and deterioration of social, economic and physical health.

The emptying of the family nest largely brings to an end the role of parent and requires that we lay aside the well-honed skills we required to raise our children. Most of us find new use for these skills as we become grandparents. The skills we developed nurturing our children can find broader use in caring for and nurturing ideas, organizations, inventions, and community improvement. We can use them to tutor children having difficulty in school, mentor youth whose future career interests are near our own, and sustain young people during illness or family crisis. Those who are grandparents of adolescents might make splendid counselors for the church youth group. Organizations like Foster Grandparents and the Retired Senior Volunteers Program provide opportunities to use parenting skills.[20]

Retirement largely brings to an end the role of worker, and we are expected to lay aside the knowledge and skills, and most of the associations, we've developed as adults. Some put their skills and knowledge to new use in second careers, often turning a hobby or special interest into a profitable business. The skills we developed in business, trade or profession can find broader use through volunteer service in a host of community agencies and organizations. Business skills are needed on the boards of directors or trustees of hospitals, schools, retirement homes, and dozens of other nonprofit businesses. Almost every denomination has a volunteer missionary program through which skills learned at work can be made available to domestic and overseas schools, hospitals, and other mission projects. Organizations like the Service Corps of Retired Executives afford opportunity for those experienced in business to mentor those just starting out.[21]

Widowhood requires that we lay aside the role of spouse, and may also bring to an end the roles of lover, confidant, and friend. Finding new outlets for the skills associated with these roles may be difficult in later life. As noted earlier, men most often remedy this loss by remarrying, but a shortage of unmarried men makes this impossible for most older women. Many community groups provide a range of opportunities for forming new friendships. Widow-to-widow groups[22] provide support and information during adjustment to loss of one's spouse. Groups like Senior Companions provide opportunity to be a friend and companion to another older person.[23]

The death of our parents usually occurs during our empty nest and retirement years, and we lose the role of child. For the first time in our lives, we are on our own. There is no one older to whom we can turn for advice, information, support, or a loan. If we are the oldest of the next generation, the death of a parent, aunt or uncle, may also bring unexpectedly the new role of head of the clan. Now we are the one to whom others of our generation, and their children, turn for information, advice, and the like.

As we settle into the years of maturity, we may find our life space shrinking, sometimes intentionally. Once the children are grown, and visits by the grandchildren have become less frequent, couples often decide that a smaller house, condominium or apartment would be easier to care for, and less expensive. Eventually some opt for the convenience of a retirement home, along with its greater security in the event of long-term illness. Smaller quarters afford less privacy, however, and retirement facilities often necessitate adjusting to tight meal schedules.

As we become accustomed to widowhood, we must adjust to living alone and shopping and fixing meals for one person. Those who live alone can in time develop a greater risk of accident, illness, and social isolation. Many dislike cooking only for themselves and in consequence fail to maintain an appropriate diet. Congregate meals, available at nearby churches and community centers, provide inexpensive nutritionally balanced meals and opportunity to meet others who live alone. Carrier Alert[24] and telephone assurance networks provide a means of summoning aid when needed by those who live alone.

GETTING IT ALL TOGETHER

Later maturity, as described in this chapter, overlaps the two final stages of generativity and maturity described by Erik Erikson.[25] While active caring for the next generation has usually ended, we may begin these years still guiding the people, ideas and things we generated. Toward the end of this stage, but before we have become infirm, we may begin putting closure on this life and readying ourselves for the next.

The recognition accorded us at retirement, combined with the love of our children and grandchildren, may enable us in later maturity to move toward the self-actualization which Maslow saw as the pinnacle of his "hierarchy of felt needs." The disengagement long thought to be desirable after age 65,[26] may even appear to be the inner feeling of detachment from the culture which Maslow found in almost all self-actualizers.[27]

The extraordinary lengthening of the years between empty nest and infirmity or death in the latter half of this century calls into question these models of life's final stage. We may achieve ego integrity or waste these years in disgust and despair, but making peace with the life we have lived until now falls short of the opportunity to live into God's purpose which these years afford us. Self-actualization resembles the hope of "getting to do what I want" which we longed for when we were young, but falls short of the self-transcendance to which Christ and his apostles call us throughout the New Testament.

Both ego integrity and self-actualization are focused upon the self. So too is much of our popular social attitude. Both Social Security and private pensions are seen as rewards for past effort. We need not report for work to receive the income they provide. We are bombarded with inducements to leisure pursuits. Idleness, once a vice, is touted as a virtue.

Instead, the transitions of later life can lead to new roles and functions, new opportunities for growth and success. All that is required of us is the creativity and imagination to see beyond the elements of loss that are part of almost every change life now brings. We need not settle for idleness, we need not be has-beens. The heroes and heroines of ancient Israel are almost all remembered and revered not for the families they raised or the careers they pursued, but for what they did late in life.[28] The same can be said for those who made the most lasting marks upon almost every society and generation since. The choice is ours whether the same will one day be said about us.

NOTES

1. Popular slogan of the 1960s, attributed to Jerry Rubin.
2. Popular television series of the late 1980s, broadcast by the American Broadcasting Company.
3. Age Discrimination in Employment Act of 1967.
4. Robert N. Butler, WHY SURVIVE? BEING OLD IN AMERICA (New York: Harper & Row, 1975), 227-228. See also Robert C. Atchley, THE SOCIAL FORCES IN LATER LIFE, Third Edition (Belmont, California: Wadsworth, 1980), 238.
5. Erik H. Erikson, CHILDHOOD AND SOCIETY (New York: W.W. Norton, 1963), 261-268; INSIGHT AND RESPONSIBILITY (New York: W.W. Norton, 1964), 124-132.
6. Erikson, CHILDHOOD AND SOCIETY, 261.
7. Erikson, INSIGHT AND RESPONSIBILITY, 124-127.
8. *Ibid.*, 131, italics in original.
9. Elisabeth Kübler-Ross, ON DEATH AND DYING (New York: MacMillan, 1969).
10. AGING AMERICA: TRENDS AND PROJECTIONS, 1987-88 Edition (Washington, DC: U.S. Senate Special Committee on Aging), 39, 60-61, 65-66, 76-77. A copy of the current edition of this publication may be obtained by writing the U.S. Senate Special Committee on Aging, Room G-31, Dirksen Senate Office Building, Washington, DC 20510, or the American Association of Retired Persons, 1909 K Street NW, Washington, DC 20049.
11. *Ibid.*, 137.
12. *Ibid.*, 23-25.
13. Timothy H. Brubaker, LATER LIFE FAMILIES (Beverly Hills: Sage Publications, 1985), 89.
14. *Ibid.*
15. *Ibid.*
16. ON DEATH AND DYING, 38-137.
17. Information about such groups can be obtained from the American Association of Retired Persons, 1909 K Street Northwest, Washington, DC 20049.

18. AGING AMERICA: TRENDS AND PROJECTIONS, 104-105, 118.

19. Carol S. Pierskalla, WHO CARES? (Valley Forge, PA: American Baptist National Ministries, 1989).

20. Look in the U.S. Government Section of your local telephone directory under ACTION, The Federal Domestic Volunteer Agency.

21. See note 20.

22. Check with a local chapter of the American Association of Retired Persons, or contact Interreligious Liaison, AARP, 1909 K Street NW, Washington, DC 20049.

23. See note 20.

24. Check with your postmaster.

25. Erik H. Erikson, IDENTITY AND THE LIFE CYCLE (New York: International Universities Press, 1959), 97-99; see also CHILDHOOD AND SOCIETY, 266-269; INSIGHT AND RESPONSIBILITY, 130-134.

26. Elaine Cumming and William E. Henry, GROWING OLD: THE PROCESS OF DISENGAGEMENT (New York: Basic Books, 1961).

27. Abraham H. Maslow, MOTIVATION AND PERSONALITY (New York: Harper & Row, 1970), 173.

28. See Chapter 3.

Chapter 7

Growing Beyond Life

Abraham breathed his last and died in a good old age, an old man and full of years, and was gathered to his people.

—Genesis 25:8 (RSV)

We spend our days, for the most part, in good health. An occasional illness puts us down for a few days now and then. We undergo surgery to repair the damage from an accident, or correct some problem, then recover in a reasonably short period of time. We develop high blood pressure or diabetes, and another chronic condition or two, but are able to control them effectively with medication or diet. We may even experience a heart attack or one or two small strokes, without much to limit behavior or alter our life style afterward. Though we have some health problems, we regard ourselves as generally in good health.

As the years wear on, following retirement, the chronic conditions take their toll. As we near our 85th birthday, we start to slow down more noticeably. As the frailty progresses, we begin to have difficulty carrying out ordinary daily tasks such as: going to the bathroom; getting dressed; fixing a meal; or going to the store without help. Or, we develop a more serious disorder, perhaps cancer, heart disease, a series of strokes that impair basic functions, or Alzheimer's disease.

Thus, we gradually enter that final stage that leads to our death. It is more common among the very old, but its onset is not determined by age. Many who are very old never enter this stage and die while they are still in generally good health, usually from an acute illness or accident. This stage is often characterized by the loss of memory and confusion popularly called senility, but many who are physi-

92

cally very frail retain full possession of their mental faculties. Instead of either *very old age* or *senility*, therefore, we have labelled this life stage simply *infirmity*.

If we define infirmity as frailty to the point of requiring help with ordinary daily activities, or the debilitating later stages of a chronic or deteriorative disease leading to death, then many of us will die without ever becoming truly infirm. The longer we live, however, the greater the probability that we will become infirm. If we live beyond age 85, one fourth of us will find ourselves in a nursing home. The odds are equally high that still living at home, we will require the help of a family member or neighbor to carry out several personal or home management activities.[1] In short, it is likely that at least one in four of us will become infirm before dying.

Our primary concern about this final period of infirmity is not whether we shall die, or when, or even how. What we most want to know is as equally important and far less academic. Who will care for us when we are too ill or too frail to care for ourselves? How can we continue to grow in faith when loss after loss comes snowballing over us toward the end of a long life? How shall we continue our discipleship when life is more a matter of receiving than giving?

ILLNESS AND LONG TERM CARE

It is often said that the old fear death far less than illness. Benjamin Franklin noted that death is as certain as taxes. Illness, however, is not certain. In our younger years, illness, although sometimes severe, has usually been brief and recovery was seldom in doubt. Illness in old age is another matter, however. It is more often chronic than acute, frequently deteriorative, and often debilitating as well. In consequence, it is not illness we fear so much as the attendant helplessness and dependence on others.

Chronic conditions are common among older adults. Among those over age 65, the most common ailments are arthritis (48 percent), high blood pressure (39 percent), hearing impairment (30 percent), heart conditions (28 percent), and orthopedic impairment (17 percent). Heart disease, cancer and stroke account for three out of four deaths among the elderly. They also account for 20 percent of doctor visits, 40 percent of hospital days, and 50 percent of all days spent in bed. A fourth of those over age 85 living in the community have difficulty performing three or more personal care tasks, and a third are unable to carry out three or more routine household chores.[2]

Improvements in health care are steadily lowering the death rates from heart disease, cancer and strokes. Research on AIDS and Alzheimer's Disease show promise of breakthroughs that may in time provide cures or even prevention. Such diseases threaten the very old, however, with both debilitation and eventual death. As noted in the previous chapter, families stretch themselves to extraordinary lengths to care for elderly relatives severely disabled by these diseases.

The presence of disabling disease is usually attended by the prospect of eventually needing the services of a nursing home. Many older people fear merely going to a hospital because people die there. Many more would rather die than go to a nursing home. In fact, most who do go there don't die, at least not at first. Few nursing homes are as bad as our worst impressions, fewer still are as good as they might be. Some have recently abandoned the use of physical and chemical restraints. Most still use physical restraints to keep the very frail from falling out of beds and chairs or deter the confused from wandering away. Physicians sometimes order medications to calm the emotionally distraught or quiet the noisy.

Aides who provide much of the care are often inadequately trained and poorly paid. Nursing homes that accept Medicare and Medicaid patients complain that reimbursement is inadequate and far less than the actual cost of care. These pages are not the place to debate the quality of nursing home care or the adequacy of reimbursement. Let it be noted, simply, that the inevitability of nursing home care is a frightening prospect for many older people. The need for that care is most likely among very old women who have been widowed and have no children, and those whose children live far away.[3] Nursing homes seem to be used as often for want of needed care at home as for the recuperative or long term medical care they were originally intended to offer.

In many communities, adult day care provides an alternative to 24-hour nursing home care. Adapted in concept from child day care, adult day care takes over during the day, while family caregivers go to work or school. Older family members are usually brought to a central location for eight to ten hours several days a week on a regular basis. Churches and religious organizations often sponsor or operate adult day care programs.

Some adult day care centers provide primarily nursing care for those requiring regular medication or physical therapy. Others provide day-long supervision and care for the very frail and those who are confused or inclined to wander. Many centers offer recreation, learning opportunities, and activities intended to reduce disorientation and confusion. Adult day care centers are as yet fewer in number than nursing homes.

A variation on adult day care also of benefit to family caregivers is respite care. The care provided is usually similar to that offered by adult day care centers. Instead of day-long care on a regular basis, respite care takes over for family caregivers to make possible an evening out, a weekend away free from responsibility, or a vacation away from home. Respite care is thus short-term but often round-the-clock. It is usually offered by a day care center or nursing home, but sometimes is separate and may be available in the family home.

THE PROCESS OF DYING

Until this century, death came at any age and most often came swiftly. Infectious diseases like tuberculosis, pneumonia and influenza were the most common killers. Farm and industrial accidents were common. Heart attacks were more often fatal than today. Deteriorative diseases like AIDS and Alzheimer's Disease were unknown, perhaps because most died first of something else. The progressive memory loss and confusion often termed senility was most often the result of a series of strokes. It was thought to be the normal consequence of old age, but wasn't often seen as life threatening.

In the United States, three out of four older persons die from heart disease, cancer or stroke. Advances in cardiac care have lowered the death rate from heart disease, but it remains the number one killer, accounting for half of all deaths among those over age 85. Deaths from cancer, especially lung cancer, continue to increase in number. Pneumonia and influenza account for relatively few deaths among the elderly, but is the cause of one in fifteen deaths among those over age 85.[4]

The very medical technologies which today save lives also sometimes prolong the process of dying. This writer is not qualified to discuss the complex issues and often conflicting viewpoints that surround the use of respirators, resuscitation procedures, and feeding tubes. Let it be noted, simply, that without their use patients would often die sooner. Some would rather be allowed to die without their aid; some fear their use even more than they fear death itself.

There are alternatives. Some physicians will honor family requests that extraordinary measures not be used, and sometimes will counsel that approach. Some will enter a Do Not Resuscitate (DNR) order on the patient's chart. When cardiac arrest occurs, however, emergency teams sometimes do not notice or honor such orders. Once life support devices have been put in use, turning them off becomes very complicated. Most physicians, nurses and hospitals find it impossible to take such action. To do so is forbidden in nearly all states, and may be construed as murder in some.

Many states have enacted legislation allowing for living wills and durable powers of attorney. These documents allow a patient, while still competent to make such decisions, to limit or forbid the use of life supports or resuscitation procedures, and to entrust to a family member or friend decisions about such matters.[5]

Hospice is a special alternative for the care of terminally ill patients, usually those with cancer, during the final weeks or months when death is certain and imminent. The concept comes from the middle ages when religious orders established places of hospitality where the suffering of the dying could be alleviated. The first modern hospice, St. Christopher's, was established in London in 1967. Its aim is to free the patient from pain and the memory and fear of pain, and to provide comfort and companionship to patients. Family members, including children, may visit at any time, except one day a week when they may not visit and need not feel guilty about it. They are also encouraged to help with the patient's care.[6] The hospice concept has spread widely throughout the U.S. and centers may now be found in most larger cities.

LOSS AND GRIEF

Loss is inevitable. It is our very nature as humans to form attachments to other people, and to places and things. Nothing in life is tied down, however; nothing is permanent. When people die we experience the pain of letting go. Every experience of leaving or being left is a little death accompanied by the same sense of loss. Only the degree of pain varies.

We experience loss throughout life, but it is particularly a feature of the later years. Our children leave home and we must let go of them. We lose the familiar role of parent. With that change, we must also give up our youth. Later we lose our jobs and must let go of the people and places associated with them. Now we must give up a major part of our identity and the roles of worker and provider, employee or boss. People who matter to us move away or die: parents, siblings, friends, husband or wife, children. If we also move to a smaller house or to retirement accommodations, we must let go of familiar friends, neighbors, surroundings, and the roots we have put down in a community.

Sometimes there are compensations for the losses during empty nest and retirement years, beginnings that offset some of the endings. These can include grandchildren, new neighbors and friends, new surroundings, new activities, new leisure pursuits, new commitments to church or civic organizations. The losses of this final stage of infirmity differ in some important ways. They are characterized by rapidity and finality, and are ever-present and cumulative.[7]

Experiences of separation and loss are common in a highly mo-·bile society, and we may even have experienced the death of a close friend or relative before middle age. Now, as the years mount up, we begin to lose others through death with increasing frequency. In addition to the loss of roles and functions, youth and identity, we now face the loss of health, mobility, control, self-reliance, autonomy, and perhaps even our very personhood. Finally, we must face the loss of the future, and of life itself.

The false gods — youth, attractiveness, intelligence, money, power, influence — all begin to fail us. Neither cosmetics nor insurance can stave off the ravages of disease and time. Nor will our faithfulness in worship, our generosity in benevolence, or our diligence in service, afford us enough chips to bargain our way out of these losses.

The experience of loss begins with our birth, when we must give up the warmth and security and total connectedness of the womb. Over the years, in addition to people, places, and things, we lose "romantic dreams, impossible expectations, illusions of freedom and power, illusions of safety" and the younger self we expected to remain forever "unwrinkled and invulnerable and immortal."[8] The myriad losses we experience throughout life are the product of attachment and separation, and provide the basis for our lifelong growth. Every loss is a little death that contains the potential for rebirth. Who and what we become is determined in large measure by the process of individuation, of separating ourselves from the people and places of our birth. We grow and develop by giving up and letting go that which is safe and familiar. The experience of loss is part of life, and is necessary because "we grow by losing and leaving and letting go."[9]

The connection between loss and growth is easier to perceive in the earlier years of life. When we are younger, leaving and letting go is part of moving on to something bigger and better. In the final months and years of our infirmity, the connection is harder to find. We do not readily see how letting go of health and the ability to care for ourselves can possibly be related to growth, how giving up autonomy and becoming dependent on others can become the basis for continued development.

Infirmity, life's final stage, is inevitably a time not only of loss but of grieving, for grief is a normal human response to loss. We are more aware of grief as an experience that follows a loss, but it can also be, and often is, in anticipation of a loss. With the coming of infirmity and the growing awareness and certainty of helplessness and death, grief is a natural reaction. As we anticipate the possible or probable loss of some bodily function, or the prospect of a future without some internal organ, intense and unexpected feelings are likely.

Elisabeth Kübler-Ross found that dying patients often worked their way slowly through denial and isolation, anger, bargaining, depression, and finally acceptance.[10] Grief is a very personal and highly individual experience. It is an unpredictable and disorderly process that usually evokes a number of intense feelings, such as numbness, emptiness, loneliness, isolation, fear and anxiety, guilt and shame, anger, sadness and despair, and physical symptoms such as pain or shortness of breath.[11] To avoid or soften grief's impact, we employ a variety of defense mechanisms. We may refuse to admit the reality of the loss (denial), convince ourselves it won't be so bad (rationalization), or overvalue that which we have lost or are about to lose (idealization). We may also overemphasize the opposite state (reaction formation), or act out an earlier stage of existence (regression).[12]

As we settle into the months or years of our infirmity, the focus of our experiences of loss, and our grief, shifts gradually from bodily functions and social relationships to life itself. At first we are aware of the loss of ability to care for ourselves, the inconvenience of depending on others for aid. The autonomy we worked so hard to attain when we were young begins to slip away. We experience again a dependence like that we knew when we were young. Then we looked forward to growing up and freeing ourselves of the influence and control of others. Now we must anticipate further decline and a greater need to be cared for. We remember expressions like "second childhood," and realize they now apply to us.

As our illness progresses, as we become more frail and in need of others' help, the probability and proximity of our death takes precedence over other sensations of loss. Finitude is a part of life. No one gets out of this life alive. Yet as a society, we conspire to deny this truth and to conceal death when it appears. Our language is filled with euphemisms that hide death's stark reality and liken it to sleeping or to a journey. We spend large sums to camouflage its visage and inter our bodies in watertight vaults that delay but cannot prevent their decay and the return of our elements to the earth from which they came.

When loved ones die we reminisce about their lives but speak little about their deaths. We mourn our loss, but beyond ritual affirmations of our resurrection faith and reassurances of their translation to the presence of God, give little thought to what death means for the one who has died. We come thus unprepared to contemplate the significance of our own impending death. Yet that is exactly what we need to do.

Like death, grief makes us uncomfortable, and we would rather avoid its presence. It is a necessary process, however, without which we cannot recover from experiences of deep loss. It's goals are: (a) that we acknowledge and express our feelings of pain and confusion at the leaving and letting go of anyone or anything of consequence in our lives; (b) that we take stock of our loss, assess its meaning for our lives, and accept its reality; (c) that we resolve the doubts and questionings that have called into question our values and shaken our faith in God; and (d) that we reorganize our life so as to get on with living.

One of the truisms of counseling is that feelings, whether or not justified, are facts. Grief that anticipates a loss has a way, therefore, of making the loss a fact. Whether or not they are warranted, we must deal with our feelings. Rationalizing or denying these feelings are not means of adjusting to loss, but a defense against them. Whether a loss has already occurred, or is anticipated, grief is the natural process for resolving it. When a loss is of great consequence, especially when it is the loss of a human life, we may need the help of others as we grieve our way back to full functioning.

Help often takes the form of intervention. Others take over the routine tasks of our life. Following a death, family and friends bring in meals, care for household chores, run errands, and generally keep things running smoothly. They can also help by protecting us from those who would take advantage of our vulnerability to sell us things we don't need and can't afford, steal from us, or even assault us physically. The same kinds of help can be equally important when we are coping with infirmity or grieving our way toward the reality of our impending death.

There is a fine line, however, between helpful intervention and a complete takeover. The purpose of assistance must not be to make us more helpless and more dependent, but to sustain our feelings of autonomy by supporting as much functional ability as we can manage. Our natural feelings of sympathy sometimes become destructive. If you always push my wheelchair, I will soon be unable to wheel it myself. I will no longer be able to get around without aid, and I will be more helpless than before. If you always feed me, I will soon be unable to feed myself. If you always speak for me, I will soon lose the ability to communicate. I will then be more helpless than I was before you set out to help me.

Beyond such practical aid, we need support to recognize and rehearse our feelings. Only by dealing with them can we work our way through them and get on with life. By listening we can enable another person to acknowledge and express feelings of loss and grief. The purpose of our listening is to express empathy for the other's feelings, and thereby lend strength and support. Empathy legitimates the other's experience and feelings. It differs from sympathy, in which we take part in the other's feelings with them. It is not helpful to cry when the other cries. It is neither necessary nor useful to document that we have felt the same by relating tales of our own loss. Just as there are limits to intervention, there must be limits to our efforts to share the other's feelings. Go easy on the comfort.

When grief follows an actual loss, encouraging the other to remember the person, place or object, is an important part of letting go. It serves to reinforce positive images and feelings associated with the memories of loss and pain. The positive feelings become a way of keeping the lost even while leaving the pain or letting it go. When loss is anticipated, remembering can still be an important adjunct to grieving. By calling up positive images and feelings associated with the role or function that is soon to be lost, or even life itself, we can ease the process of letting go. By such remembering as we come to the end of life, we accomplish that "acceptance of one's own and only life cycle as something that had to be and that, by necessity, permitted of no substitutions" which Erikson saw as the final task of life in preparation for death.[13]

Throughout life, we take part in a conspiracy of silence on the matter of death. We seldom speak of it except when someone dies, and then only in hushed tones. Despite the official assurances of our religious tradition, no one has ever returned to describe what happens after death, nor to assure us that God is truly in charge of the outcome. The unexpected death of a loved one, the accidental death of a young person, strikes us as both inexplicable and untimely. The death of others leaves us with too many unanswered doubts to permit us to go gently into the dark night of our own death.

The most important task of grieving our way toward the end of life, and that with which we may require the greatest amount of help, must be the reintegration of our faith. Definitions and descriptions of faith can be standardized for purposes of academic discussion, but it is a very personal and often very fragile thing. All of the admonitions to listen rather than talk, and go easy on the comfort, therefore apply here of even greater necessity.

"To have faith is to be sure of the things we hope for, to be certain of the things we cannot see" (Hebrews 11:1). Faith is not some inner quality some have and others don't. Faith is the inner strength we discover as we work our way through the time of uncertainty that lies between an ending and a beginning. It is the trust in God which becomes the foundation on which we build for a future we cannot see. It is the confidence that God will not leave us to make our way alone but will bring us to a new beginning fashioned especially for us. It is God's *bon voyage* gift as we embark on a journey to an uncertain destination.

GROWING UP IS HARD

We began these chapters by recalling our childhood images of growing up, our expectation that someday we would be grown up enough that we would get to do whatever we wanted to do, and be whatever we wanted to be. Along the way we discovered that others had ideas about what we should be and do, and were able to shape our lives to their expectations. We anticipated that when our children were grown and we no longer needed to work, we might at last realize our childhood hope and might finally be grown up enough to be in charge of our own lives. Whether or not we succeeded, we may find it difficult to perceive that months or years of steadily worsening infirmity can possibly be construed as continued growth and development. How can giving up people and responsibilities that filled our lives with joy, how can letting go of life itself, be growing up?

If it hasn't happened before, infirmity may finally enable us to comprehend what growing up is all about. The prospect of losing our life may finally enable us to find it. Sometimes life seems to resemble an artichoke. The outer leaves of a mature artichoke are large but tough and stringy. They are best discarded for there is little in them worth eating. As we strip away the outer leaves, we come first to smaller but meatier ones, and finally to the savory heart itself. The accelerated loss and letting go of our later years, and particularly of infirmity, can be a kind of stripping away of people, places and things that have meant little to us, and even of many that have meant a great deal, until finally we come to the heart of the matter.

The Old Testament stories of Israel's heroes and heroines, noted in Chapter 3, recall mostly how older men and women reached beyond the parameters of parenting and work in what might otherwise have been their empty nest and retirement years. We must turn to the New Testament for understanding of the possibilities in our infirmity.

Jesus calls us to let go of home and family, give up fishing and tax collecting, to follow him. He warns that we must be prepared to let go of everything non-essential.

> Foxes have holes, and birds have nests, but the Son of Man has no place to lie down and rest. . . . Let the dead bury their own dead. . . . Anyone who starts to plow and then keeps looking back is of no use for the kingdom of God.
>
> — Luke 9:58, 60, 62

In the early years of life, growing up involves stretching our horizons to take in evermore people, places and things. As we move on through empty nest and retirement, children leave home and we let go of the people, places and things that pertain to our work. We discover, hopefully, that we can live a rich and creative life with far less at our disposal than earlier seemed necessary. As we move on through the stage of infirmity, we have opportunity to discover that we can, and must, even part with life itself, but by doing so extend life beyond its present finitude. "I tell you, most solemnly, unless a wheat grain falls on the ground and dies, it remains only a single grain; but if it dies, it yields a rich harvest" (John 12:24 Jerusalem Bible). "Anyone who wants to save his life will lose it; but anyone who loses his life for my sake, and for the sake of the gospel, will save it" (Mark 8:35 Jerusalem Bible).

My deep desire is that . . . I shall bring honor to Christ, whether I live or die. For what is life? To me, it is Christ. Death, then, will bring more. . . . I want very much to leave this life and be with Christ. . . .

—Philippians 1:20-23

Were there no life, there would be no death. Were there no attachments in our life, there would be no separations. Were there no love, there would be no loss, no need for grief. We love and lose because God loves us and creates us able to love and feel pain. We live because God gives life; we let go of life in order to live more fully. We grieve over our losses in order that we may keep imperishable what we have lost. We grieve over our death to come in order that we may realize the fullness of God's gift of life.

NOTES

1. AGING AMERICA: TRENDS AND PROJECTIONS, 1987-88 Edition (Washington, DC: U.S. Senate Special Committee on Aging), 104, 118.
2. *Ibid.*, 97-110.
3. *Ibid.*, 118-119.
4. *Ibid.*, 109-110.
5. For more information, contact the Society for the Right to Die, 250 West 57th Street, New York, NY 10107. They can provide forms legally acceptable in your state for both living wills and durable powers of attorney.
6. Robert C. Atchley, THE SOCIAL FORCES IN LATER LIFE, Third Edition (Belmont, CA: Wadsworth, 1980), 204.
7. R. Scott Sullender, LOSSES IN LATER LIFE (Mahwah, NJ: Paulist Press, 1989), 16-18.
8. Judith Viorst, NECESSARY LOSSES (New York: Fawcett, 1987), 2.
9. *Ibid.*, 3.
10. Beth Kübler-Ross, ON DEATH AND DYING (New York: MacMillan, 1969).
11. Kenneth R. Mitchell and Herbert Anderson, ALL OUR LOSSES, ALL OUR GRIEFS (Philadelphia: Westminster, 1983), 61-82.
12. R. Scott Sullender, LOSSES IN LATER LIFE, 6-10.
13. Erik H. Erikson, CHILDHOOD AND SOCIETY (New York: W.W. Norton, 1963), 268.

Chapter 8

A Place to Grow In

Every man desires to live long, but no man would be old.

— Jonathan Swift

Maturity and old age are becoming almost universal human experiences. Within the past fifty years, life spans in excess of seventy years have become the norm in the United States and western Europe. Before another half century has elapsed, such long lives will be usual almost everywhere.

As our years have increased, so have the numbers of mature and older people. Because the birth rate has been simultaneously low for nearly twenty-five years, society's needs and priorities have changed. The rapid expansion of public school facilities in the 1950s and 1960s has given way to a building boom in retirement housing and longterm care facilities during the 1970s and 1980s. In almost every community, a host of activities and services are available to help older adults resolve health or financial problems, continue their education, be of service to others in difficulty, or just pass the time of day.

Awareness of these changes has spread rapidly in recent years. Feature stories about the "Graying of America" have made the pages of national magazines from ESQUIRE to U.S. NEWS & WORLD REPORT. Major daily newspapers and television network news have provided similar coverage. New books and periodicals about aging and older people appear daily. National organizations devoted to the needs and concerns of the elderly attract members by the thousands, sometimes millions. The impact on our social life has been pervasive. Few institutions have escaped the need to respond to this widespread revolution.

The lengthening of life and the consequent increase in the number of older people has not been without an impact upon the church.

Fellowship halls and parish houses once used primarily by youth and family groups now house congregate meals, recreation programs and educational activities for older people. Nursing homes and retirement complexes developed by congregations and other religious organizations house millions of older people.

One fifth to one fourth of the total membership of many denominations is now over age 65. In many congregations one half to two thirds of the membership is elderly. Rapid growth in the number of older people has not, however, led to widespread development of religious education and pastoral ministries designed specifically for older people.

Congregations often reflect society's preference for those who are young, attractive, verbal, intelligent and successful. Attitudes toward older church members are likely to be influenced more by commonly held myths and stereotypes than by knowledge of actual circumstances. Older people are often perceived as unattractive, confused, garrulous, uninteresting and dependent. Their needs are seen as a drain on limited resources that threatens other church programs. Awareness of their growing numbers often leads only to increased efforts to attract younger people to church membership.

A congregation's life flourishes or languishes according to how we nurture the faith of individuals. Much of the church's future strength depends therefore upon the quality of our ministry with older adults. Because they are a large part of the church's present membership, we must be responsive to their needs and concerns. Because they are the most rapidly growing portion of the congregation, we need their participation and their help in shaping the church's future. Because most older adults grow through the years in faith and commitment, as well as skill and experience, we need them to nurture the faith and guide the developing commitment of others.

ARGUMENTS IN FAVOR OF OLDER ADULT MINISTRY

Churches have not been entirely insensitive to this matter. National and regional church bodies have formed committees and employed staff to consider what is to be done in response to the growing numbers of older church members. Some congregations have developed activities and services for older people. A few larger churches have employed pastors for their older members. Among the arguments commonly voiced in support of greater attention to the needs and concerns of older people are the following arguments.

The "Ain't It Awful" Argument

This is the oldest and best known rationale for concern about the elderly. It provides the basis for Social Security, transportation and housing subsidies, Medicare and Medicaid. It consists largely in the widespread belief that most older people are poor, sick, destitute and alone in the world.

Growing older can bring increased difficulties. Cancer, Parkinson's Disease, and Alzheimer's Disease are frightening companions of the old. Recovery from acute illness is slower, requiring longer hospital stays, more visits to the doctor, and larger expenditures for prescription drugs. Nonetheless, most older people (72 percent) claim their health is good or excellent.[1]

Most older adults (80 percent) suffer from at least one chronic condition, and many have multiple problems. Among those over age 65, 50 percent suffer from arthritis, 39 percent from hypertension, 30 percent from hearing loss, 26 percent from heart conditions. Nonetheless, fewer than one in five (19 percent) experience any limitation in daily activities, and only four percent are severely disabled, as a result of chronic disease.[2]

Median family incomes for families headed by someone over age 65 average three-fifths ($18,236 in 1984) as much as for families headed by someone under age 65 ($29,292). One third of the elderly have cash incomes less than 150 percent of the poverty index. As a result, they lack the resources to withstand a serious financial crisis. On the other hand, poverty is far less widespread among older people than twenty-five years ago. When the federal poverty index was first used (1959), one third (35.2 percent) of all older people had incomes below that level. Today poverty affects older people (12.4 percent in 1984) at about the same rate as adults under age 65 (11.7 percent in 1984).[3]

Three out of five older women, but only one out of ten older men, are widowed. Two out of five older women, and one out of five older men, live alone. A few make the streets their home. Others live in nursing homes or "single room occupancy" hotels.

Nonetheless, three out of four older people own the homes they occupy, and four out of five older home owners have paid off their mortgages.[4] Four out of five older people have living offspring, and three fourths live in the same household or within a half hour's drive of at least one adult child. Half of the elderly report seeing one of their children within the last two days, another fourth within the last week. More than half of the help older adults receive in their homes is provided by relatives.[5]

Most older adults are relatively little afflicted with the misfortunes that form the popular image of old age. Nonetheless, the myths and stereotypes persist. Perceiving older Americans to be largely cut off from the "American Dream," we are quick to apply the "American Solution": There is nothing money can't fix.

Social Security, particularly following changes made during the 1970s, has lifted many older Americans from poverty. At the same time it has contributed to a significant reduction in the employment of older people. Age, rather than need, has become the basis for ending a lifetime of work. In 1950, almost half the elderly men stayed in the work force after age 65. Today fewer than one in five is working or looking for work. Two of every five women aged 55 to 64 is employed, but only one in twelve after age 65. Early retirement options, coupled with the availability of reduced Social Security benefits as early as age 62, have lowered employment among men aged 55 to 64 from nearly 90 percent in 1950 to less than 75 percent today.[6]

Medical benefits for the elderly have improved access to needed health services. More than a million nursing home beds have become available since the introduction of Medicare and Medicaid. Medicare, however, pays less than half the total health care bill for older people, and out-of-pocket expenditures for health care are the same today as before the introduction of Medicare and Medicaid. Older people spend almost ten percent of their before tax income for health care, compared to four percent for those aged 55 to 64.[7]

Nonetheless, older adults have benefitted from the "ain't it awful" philosophy. A wide range of publicly and charitably funded social and health services is now available to help them cope with many of the problems they encounter as they grow older. As churches have become concerned about older people's needs, they have sometimes emulated the programs typically offered by community agencies. In many cases, as a result, availability and accessibility of such services has been increased.

When a congregation offers social and health services to older people, how does it differ from other community agencies that offer the same services? When clergy administer such programs, how are they different from the social workers and public administrators who operate similar programs? Are social and health services the most important forms of ministry churches can offer older adults? These are tough questions, but they need to be asked.

The "Ain't It Wonderful" Argument

This somewhat newer approach is widely used to sell everything from fast food to fast cars. One television commercial seems to equate getting older with getting better. In another, an attractive model declares herself proud to be over forty. What appears at first to be appreciation of age turns out instead to be a marketing scheme based on the popular perception of old age as something undesirable. Getting better, or pride in being over forty, is the promised result of using hair coloring to hide the gray that is a sign of age. Recent magazine ads for facial cream have been a little more honest. Their pretty model admits no wish to age attractively; she intends to resist growing old.

Magazines, newspapers, and television programs that a few years ago reported America's graying trend, now feature 65 year old college freshmen, 75 year old marathon runners, and people starting a second, third, or fourth career at 85 or 90. Others call attention to the number of painters, writers, composers, and performers still active long after age 65, or doing their best work late in life. Churches celebrate the later life contributions of elderly members. Such individuals are presented as examples of graceful and successful aging. When interviewed, however, many protest being described as old. They, like others, seek to avoid the stigma of old age by competing with individuals many years their junior, or by engaging in activities more common among younger adults.

Some magazine articles and television reports would have us believe that older people are no longer poor, sick, and lonely. A national group promotes "equity" among the generations, arguing that older people benefit at the expense of younger age groups.

Those who hold such positions often argue that tax supported programs that serve the elderly are no longer needed. They propose eliminating or reducing public funding for Medicaid, housing assistance, legal aid, and other programs that assist primarily low income older people.

A few of the elderly have incomes large enough to be termed affluent. Others have enough disposable income to attract the attention of those who would help them spend it. The leisure, sporting goods, resort housing, and tourism industries aggressively market their products and services to this age group. A number of monthly periodicals are aimed at those age 50 and older. Some cable television services are meant primarily for them. At national conventions of aging organizations, exhibitors promote mass marketing services targeted specifically to middle and higher income older adults. Others display costly products designed to ease life in the later years.

A common variant of the "ain't it wonderful" philosophy of aging is the attitude that retirement brings exemption from duty. Organizations that rely heavily on volunteer service and leadership, including churches and synagogues, often encounter this attitude to their dismay. When asked to take on a new responsibility, individuals who have retired often reply that they have "served their turn" and it is time to recruit someone younger. Combining widespread promotion of a leisure oriented lifestyle with such a concept of exemption from duty because of age has a way of turning retirement into a bread and circuses affair.

Older adults have nonetheless benefitted from the "ain't it wonderful" attitude. Many have received long overdue recognition for the accomplishments of their later years. There is somewhat less inclination to regard older people as has-beens. Advertising increasingly features older adults as consumers and valued employees. Mandatory retirement has been outlawed.[8] Skilled older workers are encouraged to remain on the job after age 65, or called back as consultants.

When congregations celebrate the later life accomplishments of older members, do they unwittingly promote the "you're not getting older, you're getting better" outlook? When religious organizations operate retirement housing that differs little from commercially operated resort housing, can it legitimately be called a ministry? How do clergy-led tours to exotic places differ from commercially operated tours to the same places? These too are tough questions, but they also need asking.

The *"Because It's There"* Argument

This premise is similar to Sir Edmund Hilary's often quoted explanation of his urge to climb Mount Everest. Over the last fifty to seventy-five years, dramatic increases in longevity have led to spectacular increases in the number of older people in western societies. When a third of the population is over 50, and almost everyone can expect to live until 80 or 90, it is argued, we can no longer ignore those among us who are old.

From the beginning the number of older Americans has grown more rapidly than the total population. The first U.S. census in 1790 reported a total U.S. population of some four million, of whom about eighty thousand (one out of every fifty) were aged 65 or older. By 1900, the total population had multiplied 19 times, while the number over age 65 had grown by nearly 38 times. Out of about 75 million Americans, some three million (one of every twenty-five) were now over 65.

Over the last few decades, however, increases in the number of older Americans have been nothing short of startling. Since the turn of the century, the total U.S. population has increased only a little more than three times, but the number over age 65 has increased more than nine times. Now, out of some 240 million Americans, nearly 30 million (one out of every eight) are age 65 or older. In the most recent census decade (1970 to 1980), while the total U.S. population increased by 9 percent, the number over age 65 grew by 23 percent, and the number over age 85 by 67 percent![9]

Such changes are expected to continue for at least another forty years, until all of the baby boom generation, those born between 1946 and 1965, have reached age 65. By the year 2030, some 65 million Americans will be over age 65, more than three times as many as in 1970. One out of five (21.2 percent) will be in this age group. Over this same fifty year period, younger age groups are expected to grow much more slowly or not at all. Those aged 18 to 54 will remain fairly constant at 47 percent of the population, increasing in numbers from 95 million in 1970 to 143 million in 2030. Those under age 18 will increase from 70 million (1970) to only

73.5 million (2030), declining from 34 percent of the population to 24 percent.[10]

Many religious bodies report that 20 to 25 percent of their total membership is over age 65. One major Protestant group estimates that 51 percent of its membership is over age 50. In nearly half of its congregations, half or more of the membership is over age 65.[11] In consequence, congregations of every kind and size have begun to focus more attention on older adults. Denominations have begun to develop program resources and train leaders for older adult ministries.

These increases have some people worried, however. For more than twenty years the U.S. fertility rate has hovered around 1.7 to 1.8 live births per woman. This is well below the so-called standard replacement rate of 2.1 births needed to maintain a stable population that neither shrinks nor grows. If the fertility rate remains below the replacement rate for too long, there will not be enough young people to fill entry level jobs in industry and the military. In the short run, this is likely to lessen the emphasis on early retirement of older workers. In the long term, it could have serious economic consequences for the U.S. and other industrial nations.[12]

Some worry about the future of Social Security and Medicare. If the number of retired people continues to increase, and the number of workers does not rise as fast, will taxes for Social Security need to rise so high that workers have too little to show for their efforts? If the number of very old people (those over age 85) continues to rise rapidly, will their increased need for health services and longterm care bankrupt their families or send health care costs through the roof? Will these changes shortchange children, or lead to open conflict and strife between the generations?

Despite these concerns, older adults have benefitted from because-it's-there reasoning. A wide range of products and services have been developed specifically for those over age 50. Older women and men need no longer buy clothing designed for younger bodies in order to appear fashionable yet casual. Models well past age fifty or sixty regularly appear in television commercials and magazine ads. In some they still promote denture adhesives and laxatives. In others, however, they are shown starting new jobs or displaying a romantic interest in each other. In many ways, older people are now being seen in a more attractive and positive fashion than ever before.

Older people seldom vote as a bloc, yet their numbers have influenced the development and perpetuation of legislation that responds to their needs or serves their interests. The federal *Age Discrimination Act* assures that publicly funded services aid the elderly in proportion to their numbers. The *Age Discrimination in Employment Act* protects older workers against discrimination in the workplace and has eliminated compulsory retirement.

If congregations expand their program offerings for older adults, without considering the circumstances of their life or their developmental needs, are they simply bowing to the pressure of numbers? If denominations end compulsory retirement for clergy, but do not rethink their role in the church's life as pensioners, what difference will it make? If clergy pay more attention to older members because their contributions keep the church going, but do not nurture their spiritual growth and call them to new discipleship, will that keep the church from dying? These are very hard questions, but asking them is important.

AN ARGUMENT FROM DESIGN

A better rationale for the church's role in older adults' lives is what might be called *The Argument from Design*. It consists of those propositions raised in earlier chapters. We are meant to live much longer than necessary to carry out the basic adult functions of parenting and work. The absence of roles for the active years following the empty nest and retirement leads us to ask why we must grow older. Many of the key actors in our faith history are remembered most for what they did late in life. It was their readiness to answer God's call that enabled them to play a significant role in the community's life.

Most important of all, we need a reason for growing older, and a context to do it in. Having grown older, we need something to do that is at least as significant as rearing children and carrying out some trade or career. God's will for creation includes the purpose for our growing older. God's call includes what we are to do in our later years. In establishing the church, God has provided a place in which to discover God's will and hear God's call. Most of all, in the church God has created a context in which to grow up and grow older.

The New Testament is rich in images of the church,[13] but the term by which it is most often called is *ecclesia*. It was a common term in first century Greek, connoting an assembly or community *called together* for some specific *purpose*.

The church is a chosen people. It consists of those called together by God in Christ (Romans 8:28, I Corinthians 1:9, Colossians 3:15). "You did not choose me; I chose you. . . . " (John 15:16). Out of grace (Romans 11:5), God chose the church for his own (Colossians 3:12, I Thessalonians 1:4). Those who are poor God chose "to be rich in faith and to possess the kingdom which he promised to those who love him" (James 2:5).

The call to be God's people has a purpose. As God's chosen people, we are to do God's work in the world. "I chose you and appointed you to go and bear much fruit, the kind of fruit that endures" (John 15:16). We are called out of darkness "to proclaim the wonderful acts of God" (I Peter 2:9). From the number of times three key terms appear, it is clear that the work God calls the church to do in the world consists of (1) *kerygma*, proclamation, preaching; (2) *koinonia*, community, fellowship, participation, sharing; and (3) *diakonia*, ministry, service.

It is not for acts of preaching and proclamation alone that the church is called together but for the content of the *kerygma*. This is the good news of the Kingdom of God (Matthew 24:14,[14] Acts 20:24-25, 28:31). It is the call to repentance, uttered first by John the Baptizer (Matthew 3:1), then by Jesus himself (Matthew 4:17), and later by Christ's disciples (Matthew 6:12). The *kerygma* is an intensely personal message about what God in Christ has done. It is the irrepressibly joyous witness of one cured of a dread skin disease (Mark 1:45), another freed of the influence of demonic forces (Mark 5:20), a third to whom speech and hearing have been restored (Mark 7:36). At the same time it is the proclamation of a new world order, of good news to the poor, of liberty to the captives and freedom to the oppressed (Luke 4:18-19).

The *kerygma* is the good news that the right time (*kairos*) is at hand (Matthew 10:7), that Jesus of Nazareth is the long-awaited messiah (Acts 8:5), the offspring of God (Acts 9:20). It is a word of judgment (Acts 10:42) and a call to turn away from sin (Matthew 12:41), the assurance of God's forgiveness (Luke 24:47) and of healing (Luke 9:2). Though to the worldly-wise it seems foolish, to believers the *kerygma* is the promise of salvation (I Corinthians 1:21). The basis of our faith (I Corinthians 15:11-14), the *kerygma* is to be proclaimed to all people (Mark 13:10) for God bars none from its promises (Acts 10:34-43).

The *kerygma* is proclaimed to older people and through them. To Abraham at age 100 and to Sarah, childless in her old age, was born a son (Genesis 18:1-14, 21:1-7). God promised,

> I will make my covenant with you and give you many descendants. . . . Your wife Sarah will bear you a son and you will name him Isaac. I will keep my covenant with him and with his descendants for ever. It is an everlasting covenant.
>
> — Genesis 17:2,19

To Zechariah and Elizabeth, another childless older couple (Luke 1:18), God caused a son to be born who would "go ahead of the Lord to prepare his road for him, to tell his people that they will be saved by having their sins forgiven" (Luke 1:76-77). To Simeon and Anna, both very old, God revealed the infant Jesus as the Messiah for whom they and others waited (Luke 2:25-38).

The *kerygma* is a call to *koinonia*, to fellowship, community, participation, and sharing. From the beginning, those who believed gathered frequently (Acts 1:14). "They spent their time in learning from the apostles, taking part in the fellowship, and sharing in the fellowship meals and the prayers" (Acts 2:42). *Koinonia* is more than a gathering of like-minded folk. To be in the company of believers is to have fellowship with Christ (I Corinthians 1:9), to participate in his suffering (Philippians 3:10, I Peter 4:13). "The cup we use in the Lord's Supper and for which we give thanks to God: when we drink from it, we are sharing [*koinonia*] in the body of Christ" (I Corinthians 10:16). When we have fellowship with Christ, we "have fellowship with one another, and the blood of Jesus . . . purifies us from every sin" (I John 1:7).

The *koinonia* is an inclusive fellowship. Membership comes by faith only. Every day God adds to our number those who are being saved (Acts 2:47). No one who believes is excluded (Acts 10:34-43), not Jew or Gentile, not slave or free, not woman or man (Galatians 3:28). From the beginning older people have been part of the Christian fellowship (Titus 2:2-5). Older men (*presbyteroi*) were among the earliest leaders (I Timothy 5:17, James 5:14, I Peter 5:1-5). Imprisoned for preaching and teaching the faith, as an old man (*presbytes*) Paul continued to be a spiritual leader (Philemon 8-10).

More is at stake than simple readiness to receive whoever comes. To have fellowship with other believers is to comprehend more deeply the blessings we have through Christ (Philemon 6). "*Koinonia* is not experienced without sensitivity about injustices and damaging inequities, and the efforts to redress them. Neither is *koinonia* possible while disadvantaged and politically weak members remain passive and even apathetic about their depressed condition."[15]

From the beginning, Christians shared their belongings with the needy, opened their homes to strangers (Acts 2:44, Romans 12:13), and shared each other's sufferings (Hebrews 10:32-34). "It is as if one said that the saints are gathered into the society of Christ on the principle that whatever benefits God confers upon them, they should in turn share with another."[16] The offering Paul gathered, to help the poor Christians in Jerusalem, became for him the symbol of the *koinonia* in which Christians share. The churches in Macedonia "were extremely generous in their giving even though they are very poor. . . . First they gave themselves to the Lord, and then, by God's will they gave themselves to us as well" (II Corinthians 8:2,5).

Koinonia thus leads to *diakonia*, ministry and service. The term connotes many different kinds of assistance to others. The servants who refilled the jars at the Cana wedding (John 2:5,9), Martha (Luke 10:40, John 12:2), Peter's mother-in-law (Matthew 8:15), the women who followed Jesus (Matthew 27:55), and the angels who tended Jesus after the temptations (Matthew 4:11), all engaged in *diakonia*. Paul (Romans 11:13), Barnabus (Acts 12:25), Mark (II Timothy 4:11), Timothy (Acts 19:22), Onesiphorus (II Timothy 1:18), Onesimus (Philemon 13), and the prophets who announced Christ's coming (I Peter 1:12), were all *diakonos*, servants.

Jesus made clear that service (*diakonia*) to others is central to the life of the *koinonia*. He said that he came not to be served but to serve (*diakoneo*, Matthew 10:28). As the disciples gathered for the Last Supper, Jesus laid aside his garments, took up a basin and towel, and washed their feet (John 13:1-20). This was an act ordinarily performed by a servant. He made clear that in the Kingdom of God, greatness is achieved through service (Matthew 20:26, 23:11). Those who feed the hungry, give drink to the thirsty, receive strangers into their homes, clothe the naked, care for the sick, and visit those in prison, will "possess the kingdom which has been prepared for [them] ever since the creation of the world" (Matthew 25:34-36).

Many of the infirm elderly, and some of the mature, are clearly among those Jesus calls us to serve. The circumstances of life have improved greatly for many older people, yet severe needs exist among a large number of the elderly. Social security benefits often are not enough to provide shelter and heat, needed medications, plus enough to eat. Older people sometimes outlive all of their immediate family and become strangers in an impersonal society. Sometimes they are ashamed of worn and faded, out-of-style clothing and, as though naked, avoid other people. Many suffer from chronic and painful diseases and take longer than younger people to recover from acute illnesses. Others are literally imprisoned by the physical frailty or mental confusion brought on by heart disease, strokes, or Alzheimer's Disease. The well-being of older people, especially widows, was one of the early church's first concerns (Acts 6:1, James 1:27). The *diakonia* to which the church is today called clearly includes efforts to respond to such pressing human needs.

Mature and older Christians often engage in *diakonia* as well as receive it from others. In later life many suffer hunger, isolation and illness, but many more are healthy and active. Having finished rearing their children, mature adults often devote large amounts of time to serving others. Later, having retired from job or career, some engage in fulltime *diakonia*, serving with the Peace Corps or as volunteer church workers. *Diakonia* can even be the concern of the infirm. "Even with failing eyesight or impaired hearing, in a hospital bed or wheel chair, day or night, for as long as God grants us clear minds, we can pray."[17] In a truly inclusive *koinonia*, mature and older adults will participate fully in *diakonia*, both serving and being served.

NOTES

1. AGING AMERICA: TRENDS AND PROJECTIONS, 1985-86 Edition, U. S. Senate Special Committee on Aging, 84-108.

2. *Ibid.*, 86-89.

3. *Ibid.*, 55-57, 67.

4. *Ibid.*, 111, 116.

5. CHARTBOOK ON AGING IN AMERICA, 1981 White House Conference on Aging, 104-107.

6. AGING AMERICA, 76-77.

7. *Ibid.*, 4, 63, 105.

8. AGE DISCRIMINATION IN EMPLOYMENT ACT, 1986 Amendments.

9. AGING AMERICA, 12.

10. *Ibid.*; CHARTBOOK ON AGING IN AMERICA, 5.

11. Presbyterian Panel, October 1980.

12. Cf. Ben J. Wattenburg, "The Birth Dearth: Dangers Ahead?" in U. S. NEWS & WORLD REPORT (Volume 102, Number 24), June 22, 1987, 56-63.

13. See Paul S. Minear, IMAGES OF THE CHURCH IN THE NEW TESTAMENT (Philadelphia: Westminster, 1960).

14. Where parallel passages appear in the synoptic gospels, only one is cited.

15. J. Robert Nelson, "The Inclusive Church" in THE CHRISTIAN CENTURY (Volume 102, Number 6), February 20, 1985, 184.

16. John Calvin, INSTITUTES OF THE CHRISTIAN RELIGION, translated by Ford Lewis Battles (Philadelphia: Westminster, 1960), 1014.

17. Catherine Brandt, STILL TIME TO PRAY (Minneapolis: Augsburg, 1983), 9.

Chapter 9

Enabling Older People to Grow

Then we shall no longer be children, carried by the waves and blown about by every shifting wind. . . . Instead, by speaking the truth in love, we must grow up in every way to Christ, who is the head.

—Ephesians 4:14-15

Just as our lives resemble plays, so the church resembles the theater. The similarity has little to do, however, with church and theater buildings. These are only meeting houses adapted to the needs of the groups who use them. The theater is people—a company drawn together by commitment to drama as a form of art, and by the call to be creative. A church is also people—a community drawn together by faith in Jesus Christ as savior and sovereign, and by the call to serve others in Christ's name.

The theater provides the milieu within which some write and others perform plays amid settings that emulate the daily world. From the theater people draw both knowledge and inspiration. Its traditions nurture their creativity and challenge their artistry. In much the same way, the church provides the milieu within which Christians create and act out their real-life plays. From the church we receive not only inspiration and knowledge, but also love and justice. Its traditions and rituals nurture our spiritual growth and discipline our servanthood.

Every individual is at once playwright and player. Every congregation is both acting company and audience. Within this context, the playlike dimensions of our life—the series of acts, the scene changes, the offstage events, the tragedy and the comedy — become significant moments (*kairoi*) for ministry. How the congregation and the individual interact at these moments greatly influences the shape of each person's life.

IN SEARCH OF A PREMISE

Until quite recently, most people died without ever reaching old age. Today, most people born in this country live well past age 65. As a result, the number of older people is increasing faster than the total population. Surrounded by more and more older people, we have become increasingly aware of the problems that often accompany the later years. In response, communities have created agencies and organizations to help older adults deal with their problems, but many of their needs remain unmet.

Community agencies usually begin with some concept of what constitutes an acceptable life style for older people. From that they develop a range of services intended to narrow the gap between individual experience and the organization's ideal. Title I of the Older Americans Act, for example, provides such a concept. It affirms that older people should enjoy adequate income, physical and mental health, suitable housing, opportunity for employment, and the like.[1] In nearly every community, services for older people such as senior centers and congregate and home-delivered meals are organized and funded under subsequent parts of this Act.

The number of older church members is growing too, and some congregations have begun to look for ways to respond to their needs. The concepts which guide a congregation as it builds its ministry with older adults will, out of necessity, be somewhat different from the foundation on which most community agencies build their programs of services for older people.

Abraham Maslow observed that human needs fall largely into a hierarchy of five levels: physiological, safety, belongingness and love, esteem, and self-actualization.[2] He believed the body's needs for food and fluids are the most innately powerful, and when chronically unsatisfied, push all other needs into the background. Maslow also believed that when one level of need is regularly satisfied, it becomes less powerful, causing the next "higher" need to be more keenly felt. In this fashion, as the individual achieves satisfaction of successive levels of felt need, self-actualization eventually emerges as the strongest force.

Maslow's behavioral model is widely used by service delivery agencies and is initially attractive as an organizing principle for older adult ministry. Most human needs seem at first to fall neatly into one or another of its well-articulated categories. The recognition that some needs are more powerful than others helps us understand why achievement, respect, love, even security, can become meaningless in the face of extreme physical deprivation. An individual's needs are not easily discerned by another, however, and it is one's *felt* needs that influence behavior. Moreover, personal experience does not always neatly match theory. Marginal deprivation in several areas at the same time may be more common than severe deprivation in any one level.

This approach seems also to lack an adequate understanding of individual spiritual needs. Maslow's self-actualizers are attractive. They are comfortable with reality, accepting of self and others, spontaneous and natural, autonomous and creative, capable in interpersonal relations, and able to distinguish good from evil.[3] Nevertheless, they fall short of the potential to which we are called. Humans are to have communion with God; we are to care for God's creation and its inhabitants. The needs Maslow describes are, by contrast, self-serving. There is little room for altruism, even less for faith grounded in the *kerygma*, nurtured in *koinonia*, and fulfilled in *diakonia*.

What the church attempts with older adults must be based on different grounds. No separation of secular from sacred, or body from spirit is intended here. The components of a congregation's older adult ministry may, in fact, be quite similar to the services a community agency offers older people. No disparagement of the efforts of "secular" organizations is intended. Community agencies begin with an awareness of human need and want and try to remedy what they find. The value of their services lies in their success in achieving that goal.

In an earlier book, I suggested that older adult ministry be organized in terms of three progressive levels of need:

Preventive

> . . . those 60 and over whose major limitations, imposed on them by society, prevent them from being just as self-sufficient as any other adults in the population;

Maintenance

> . . . those 60 and over who have been limited similarly, but who have begun to accept exclusion as "natural" and to limit their own activities to conform with this "reality"; and

Protective and Supportive

> . . . those 60 and over with "real" limitations — i.e., those imposed by social, physical, emotional or psychological handicaps, which may or may not have resulted from the natural aging process.[4]

The *preventive* ministry proposed was essentially pre-retirement education. Intended for those in middle-age, its purpose was to help them accomplish the transition from work to leisure, accept the limitations of old age, and develop new interests through continuing education. The *maintenance* ministry suggested made use primarily of recreation, outreach and in-home services to prevent or delay institutionalization of the old. The *protective and supportive* ministry described was concerned with those no longer able to care for themselves. It was understood to be primarily custodial and provided primarily by public and private long term care institutions.

These approaches were flawed as well. The perception of old age as a time of inevitable decline made it difficult to see other possibilities. The *prevention* effort was concerned mostly with adaptation while *maintenance* focused its energy on holding the line. *Protection and support* were not differentiated from merely warehousing the old. The purpose of these efforts was largely to help people get through old age with as little discomfort as possible. Little effort was directed toward challenging or changing social practices that discourage older people from useful activity. There was little expectation that older adults would continue to grow in faith or seek new opportunities for discipleship. Such an older adult ministry would differ little from other community services to older people.

The church, like many community agencies, *is* concerned about human suffering. God calls us to a ministry with very broad parameters—judgment and forgiveness, repentance and salvation, justice and an end to poverty and oppression. Forgiveness and salvation are universal human needs from which age affords no exemption. Millions of older people are poor, millions more oppressed by social customs that devalue their capabilities and debase their worth as human beings. Ministry among older people must therefore include the good news (*kerygma*) of redemption and justice, and efforts (*koinonia* and *diakonia*) to alleviate older people's most pressing wants and to correct social injustices so that older people will no longer suffer from want and injustice.

Nonetheless, in its ministry with older people, the church has an agenda different from the community agency. All ministry must always find its rationale in our best understanding of God's purpose. Our concern for older people should be no exception.

The church's mandate comes from God. Its goal is the same as God's goal for individuals—to know God and to reveal God to others, to nurture and care for what God has made, to become coworkers with Christ, and to seek the creative opportunities in life's every moment. The church that strives to carry out God's purpose in the world is called to a ministry that includes, but is not limited to, alleviating human suffering. If we begin by assessing individual needs, and design ministry solely to meet those needs, we subordinate love and justice to freedom from suffering. "Our highest goal," writes Dorothy Soelle, is then "to be free of suffering, to become free of it and remain free of it right up to the moment of death." That, she believes, "is only of secondary value and is not the goal Jesus Christ strove for."[5]

The church's ministry with older adults naturally includes efforts to alleviate suffering, correct injustice, and reach out to those who have become isolated. These efforts must not, however, become an end in themselves. Suffering, injustice and isolation prevent older people from carrying out God's purpose. Older adult ministry is concerned ultimately with enabling older people to grow continually in faith and discipleship. God calls each of us to seek the creative opportunities in life's every moment. The church's efforts to remedy the troubles that too often accompany later life ought, therefore, to free older people to seek new uses for the skills and experience accumulated over a lifetime.

Being grown up is not something that comes automatically with attainment of adulthood and the completion of formal education, nor once the children are grown and job or career have ended. To view maturity as something that occurs as a matter of course after the clock has ticked a certain number of times is to be content with a *chronos* view of human development. Being "grown up" is an issue of timing (*kairos*) and has to do with discerning God's will, of perceiving God's call at each stage, each transition, and determining what my response will be *for this time* in my life.

For the believer, being grown up cannot be simply a matter of getting to do what I want after I've done all that others expect me to do. Being grown up means discerning and saying "Yes!" to God's particular call for my life for this time and place.

In Chapter 2, I proposed that older people are called to carry out God's purpose for creation. Made in God's likeness, they are to know God and to reveal God to others. Called to nurture and care for what God has made, they are to become co-workers with Christ. Freed of time's clock-like constraints, they are to seek the creative opportunities in life's every moment. It is not enough, therefore, to organize the church's ministry around some scheme for assessing individual needs. Older people's place in the church's life must measure up to a more demanding criterion: *the church's ministry enables older adults to carry out God's purpose for their lives.*

THE SHAPE OF PASTORAL NURTURE

Older adult ministry, if it is to meet such a test, must be grounded in something like the "argument from design" set forth in Chapter 5. Such a ministry with older adults will be aptly termed *pastoral nurture*. It will commit the church to be a place where growth in faith and discipleship is lifelong. It will deal seriously with a life span far longer than needed to complete parenthood and career. It will strive to empower older adults to be fully part of those people who know themselves to be called by God (*ecclesia*). It will engage them in telling forth God's good news (*kerygma*), fellowship based on the sharing of all God's gifts (*koinonia*), and waiting upon God through the service of others (*diakonia*).

Such a ministry with older adults will be firmly rooted in the congregation's life and under the leadership of its pastor. The congregation will understand itself as neither a voluntary association of the like-minded nor a private club serving only the interests of its dues-paying members. It will be a community of called out people (*ecclesia*). Similarly, the pastor will relate to the congregation's older members neither as a servant for hire nor as an executive secretary who carries out the wishes of the organization's members, but as a prophet who, as we age, calls us and empowers us to boldly go where few have gone before.

The congregation's older adult ministry will be both *holistic* and *enabling*. It will deal with the whole person, warts and all, and will shun artificial distinctions between spiritual and physical needs, and draw no boundaries between religious and secular concerns. Moreover, it will enable us to reach for new dimensions of life as we grow older, recognizing that those whom we admire most as examples of grace-filled aging are those who now strive toward horizons more distant than those that beckoned when they were younger.

The pastoral nurture of older adults will be *proactive* in nature. It will be characterized by an intentionality rooted in God's call to each of us. Such a concept of pastoral nurture will affirm that neither age nor infirmity separates us from that love of God which empowers creation and all its inhabitants to be about God's purpose throughout life. It will therefore enable each individual to continue to grow spiritually throughout life, and will reiterate, at each of life's transitions, Christ's call to follow where he leads.

The pastoral nurture of older adults will, at the same time, be *reactive* in nature. It will be characterized by sensitivity to whatever prevents people from responding to God's call. Such a concept of pastoral nurture will recognize how readily the circumstances of our lives disable us as we grow older. It will therefore hold out both fellowship and assistance to each one isolated by loss, illness or infirmity. It will care for and support each one caught up in crisis or transition, and press for changes in policies and practices that idle and sideline people because of age or incapacity.

In dealing with older adults, pastoral nurture will be *sensitive to the differences among the generations*, yet will not unduly segregate people because of age. It will be aware that the interests of those whose children are grown have become different from the concerns of those whose children are still at home. It will be attuned to the differing issues facing those who have left the world of work and those who remain there. Most of all, it will not confuse the concerns of the infirm and dependent with those who are active and daily involved in congregation and community. It will be aware, as well, that the concerns of the active elderly may differ from those of adult children caring for frail or chronically ill parents.

The pastoral nurture of older adults will, above all, be *developmental* in nature. The concept of pastoral nurture is applicable to all ages within the church's fellowship. So too should be our concern for individual development in matters of faith and the knowledge of God. At no age are we privileged to consider that we have arrived in our understanding of what God calls us to be, or what God expects of us. The pursuit of deeper understanding, and of deeper faith, is a lifelong undertaking.

In dealing with older adults, the concept of pastoral nurture recognizes that development is normal throughout the life span. Blocking, neglecting, or short-circuiting development is abnormal. For that matter, the same attitude ought to obtain toward the experience of aging. Growing older is part of life. Pretending that it is not so, or seeking to prevent or conceal normal aging, is inappropriate behavior. If those two assumptions are accepted, then aging will be the equivalent of development, and vice versa.

Development doesn't happen by accident, however, it must be intentional. Growth is not automatic, nor will it occur in a vacuum. If the proper nutrients are not available, growth is stunted. If the environment is not conducive, growth is aborted. If the congregation is to be an effective environment for growth in faith and discipleship, we must recognize that adults learn only what they perceive a need to learn. An appeal to learning for learning's sake is seldom effective. Growth and development must have some discernible end.

The developmental end toward which pastoral nurture urges us must be something more, however, than the goal set forth in Erik Erikson's early speculations about life's eighth stage. The "ego integrity" he described is backward-looking. Anticipating death, the individual is to be concerned primarily with putting closure on life through "acceptance of one's one and only life cycle" as "the accidental coincidence of but one life cycle with but one segment of history. . . . "[6] The "wisdom" which is to be the "virtue" of this final stage, is largely *"detached concern with life itself, in the face of death itself."*[7] Such a goal is not in harmony with a commitment to enable older adults to continue to carry out God's purpose for their lives.

Carl Jung points us toward a more usable goal for pastoral nurture.

> A human being would certainly not grow to be seventy or eighty years old if this longevity had no meaning for the species to which he belongs. The afternoon of human life must also have a significance of its own and cannot be merely a pitiful appendage to life's morning.

The morning's concerns belong to nature, to individual development, the pursuit of worldly concerns, and the rearing of children, but culture lies beyond nature. "Could by any chance culture be the meaning and purpose of the second half of life?"[8]

In Jung's challenge, writes Paul Tournier, lies the call "towards a more complete human fulfillment" in the second half of life.[9] In response to Jung's question, Eugene Bianchi takes as a basic theme: "Those in elderhood are summoned to fuller participation in the great concerns of humanity."[10] This appeal, that later life be devoted to the transformation of culture, can provide the basis on which to create an older adult ministry that fully engages older people in *kerygma, koinonia,* and *diakonia.*

How to understand the relationship between Christianity and civilization is an enduring problem. In his classic study, H. Richard Niebuhr concluded that no easy answer can be found, yet "we must go farther, and arrive at a conclusion.''[11] If Jesus Christ can be the transformer of culture,[12] and we are called to be co-workers with Christ, then the development of the individual believer, beyond the limits of life's morning, into one who works for the transformation of society is an appropriate goal for the pastoral nurture of older adults.

Finally, pastoral nurture should be both *deliberate* and *contractual*. It ought to bear some resemblance to the case management used by social workers to assist older people in making effective use of the wide range of service provider agencies found today in most communities.

Spiritual growth is too important to be left to either whim or chance. As with children and youth, the spiritual development of adults needs direction. Too often we are left with inadequate resources and little sense of direction. We need from time to time, and especially in the midst of crisis or transition, to hear God's call afresh and be challenged to set new directions for our discipleship.

At the same time, pastoral nurture must not be manipulative. No matter how careful or disciplined our study of scripture and theology, we ought never presume to control in what direction another's life ought to develop so as to be faithful to God's call. But we can contract with individuals to work with them in seeking new understanding and discerning new directions for their discipleship. This caveat is particularly important in ministry with those who have become infirm and dependent upon others, and with their families. Our ability to assist them will be considerably enhanced if we have earlier established an agreement about pastoral nurture that is both understood and welcomed.

A KIND OF CASE MANAGEMENT

The concept of pastoral nurture bears some similarities to the case management provided for the elderly and their families through community agencies. Case management usually refers to the planning and coordinating of services to a client by a variety of community agencies. Its purpose is to make sure that the individual receives all of the services needed and to avoid any duplication of services. In the case of an older person, case management is often used to help an individual continue to live at home and avoid the necessity of entering a long-term care institution.

As provided by an agency's social workers, case management usually includes:

- case finding — discovering those individuals who need help,
- prescreening — determining whether the individual can benefit from case management,
- intake — initiating a mutually acceptable relationship with the client,
- assessment — determining the client's need for services,
- goal setting — agreeing with the client about what can be accomplished by case management,
- care planning — determining what services will be provided to the client,
- capacity building — helping the client work toward greater ability to care for him- or herself,
- implementation — providing or securing the services listed in the care plan,
- monitoring — checking progress toward agreed-upon goals,
- termination — ending case management when goals have been achieved,
- follow-up — keeping the door open for providing further services should the client need or want them.[13]

Case management serves a number of important purposes. Case managers help individuals determine what services they need, help them find and secure those services, act as their advocates with agencies that provide or reimburse the cost of services, and thus help individuals adapt to change, loss and decreasing resources so as to maintain their ability to function autonomously for as long as possible. Most of all, case management "help[s] people make informed decisions based upon their abilities, available resources and their personal preferences."[14]

Pastors need not become social workers and case managers. Pastoral nurture can, however, hope to achieve somewhat similar purposes, and can employ similar approaches to dealing with members of the congregation. Ministers, and lay workers engaged in pastoral ministry, can help individuals take stock of their lives, understand current transitions, and assess personal needs, while setting and working toward goals for spiritual growth and discipleship.

In place of case finding, we would seek to create a climate in which the norm would be helping each other meet personal needs and work through life's transitions, growing together in spirit and in discipleship. This is what is meant by the term *proactive* used earlier in this chapter. Each of life's transitions would be seen as an occasion for study and reflection to discern what we are called to do and be in the next act or scene. Each experience of loss or need would become opportunity to discover the resources to cope within ourselves, each other, our faith, and in God.

In place of prescreening, we would find ways to take note of life experiences that present opportunities for pastoral nurture. One way of doing this, the use of liturgical rites of passage, is discussed later in this chapter.

Intake might take the form of negotiated relationships which have as specific purposes responding to each other's needs or supporting each other during transition or crisis. Among the traditional methods for accomplishing such ends are retreats, prayer cells, and house churches. Establishing relationships for pastoral nurture can take either of two basic forms: (a) one-to-one relationships or (b) intentional groups.

Spiritual direction, personal counseling, and case management are common examples of one-to-one relationships. Case management employs the skills listed above. Personal counseling employs listening and feedback to help individuals sort their way through periods of crisis or transition or resolve problems. Spiritual direction usually includes reflection, learning of arcane disciplines, study of scripture and devotional literature, meditation and prayer. In each approach, one person presents a need for help or guidance, another makes available knowledge and access to resources and helps the first develop and pursue a plan for attaining desired ends. In some cases it may be desirable for a pastor to undertake one-to-one relationships with an individual whose needs are complex or whose spiritual pilgrimage requires expertise usually found only with a theological education. More often, intentional small groups will afford a better method of attaining the desired ends.

So-called "support groups" lend themselves particularly to this use. Using methods pioneered by Alcoholic Anonymous, these groups bring together individuals around a common concern, such as adjusting to widowhood, or caring for a family member with Alzheimer's Disease. Sometimes led by a professional counselor, more often drawing only on their own experience, group members share insights into their common concern and information about sources of help and provide each other with moral support during trying times. While more often used to aid those coping with a transition or family problem, support groups can also be used to foster growth in spiritual knowledge and discipline.

Assessment would proceed along the lines suggested throughout this book. Instead of measuring the shortfall between present reality and some concept of the good life, we would strive to discern what God has in mind for our lives, especially to what we are called within each of life's successive transitions, always seeking to understand the potential for growth present in each of life's experiences.

Goal setting should be a central characteristic of pastoral nurture, as it is of case management. In most congregations, the spiritual growth of children and young people is structured by whatever religious education process and curriculum is employed. Once we become adults, however, spiritual growth often becomes aimless and haphazard. Experience passes by unexamined, and we miss opportunities for testing our faith, for growing in spirit, and for re-examining the dimensions of our discipleship. Too often, we arrive at some major transition or crisis with a half-formed faith ill-suited to the occasion.

If you don't know where you want to go, any road will do. Life is too precious to be undertaken on such a basis. We ought, throughout the years, employ scripture, meditation and prayer, to discern the goals to which God calls us and strive to make them our own. Few will find it easy to accomplish this alone; most will benefit from the mutual support and shared insights made possible with another or with a group.

Once goals have been established, we must plan how to attain them. Since few of us possess all the resources needed for our spiritual growth, or simply to make our way through life, we would benefit from a one-to-one relationship with another or from membership in a group which shares our intentions. Our faith has been likened to one beggar showing another where to find bread. In just such fashion do we nurture each other in the faith, just so do we help each other over life's hurdles.

As with case management, capacity building is an important part of pastoral nurture. In case management, the aim is to enable the individual to maintain a functional level of autonomy as long as possible, and thus avoid dependence and the need for institutional care. In pastoral nurture, the aim should be to move from spiritual novice to seasoned disciple, as well as maintain the capacity to cope with life's transitions and crises.

Plans are worth little unless they are carried out. Here, too, we will benefit from a relationship with a mentor-counselor, or a support group. Groups that help each other carry out weight loss plans afford an apt model. When goals and plans are shared, and jointly owned by a group or by partners, our commitment to each other, or to the group, helps us remain faithful to our plans.

Monitoring is also important. On the one hand, if we cannot tell how we are doing, we will soon lose heart. If there is no way to measure progress, goals and plans may need to be revised. On the other hand, awareness that we are moving steadily toward our goals encourages us to keep moving. And, as we near one goal, we become ready to discern and claim a more distant one, thus moving always toward the ultimate prize (Philippians 3:14).

In all such supportive and nurturing relationships there exists the potential of harmful dependency. Teachers and counselors who know their limits bring to an end their relationships with students or clients who have progressed as far as they can lead them. Just so, relationships with spiritual counselors and support groups must eventually come to an end. When the individual has attained the goals set for the relationship, when the crisis that initiated the relationship has ended, when the transition has been completed, it is time to move on.

When moving away from a supportive, nurturing relationship, it is important that the door be left open for re-entering the group or renegotiating the one-to-one relationship. As time passes, new needs emerge, new transitions occur, and the need for structure and discipline returns.

Supportive relationships can be employed for many legitimate purposes. It is important, therefore, to return here to the premise stated earlier in this chapter. As a form of ministry with older adults, pastoral nurture must meet this test; *the church's ministry enables older adults to carry out God's purpose for their lives.*

RITUAL AS A FORM OF NURTURE

Worship is the central form of the church's ministry. It is, therefore, the arena in which pastoral nurture will most often be experienced and in which its functioning can most readily be exemplified.

At the heart of our worship lie traditional rites and sacraments. Repeating words and actions often first used centuries ago, they focus on our relationship with God, and on the basics of our existence — food and drink, family relationships, and social status. Dramatically and powerfully, the church's rituals affirm the significance of human events. Older people's participation in the life of the church must therefore meet this additional criterion: *The church's liturgy enables older people to accomplish and celebrate life's transitions.*

Society's rituals serve every kind of cultural, social, political and economic purpose. Through repetition of familiar word and action, they evoke our cultural memory and give meaning to contemporary events. In similar fashion, the church's sacraments and rites evoke our faith memory and point to the theological meanings in our everyday human experience. Rooted in the "tendency of living creatures to repeat their actions and thereby re-experience the accompanying emotion . . . [they] provoke the repetition of a given religious attitude which can be shared by all taking part in the rite."[15] The church's rituals are the scripts which link God's revelation to our daily lives and call forth our response.

Transition rituals, often called *rites of passage,* interpret the events which ring up the curtain on life's successive acts. They "mark the critical moments in the life career of the individual, particularly those of birth, puberty, marriage, and death."[16] Rites of passage give direction to our lives by celebrating the successful completion of one era, and setting out a road map for the next. Generation after generation, such rituals preserve and pass on our cultural traditions about the significance of life.

Rites of passage tell us who we are and what we are to do. They tell others what to expect of us, and how to behave toward us. Like the paragraphs at the beginning of each act, in which the playwright describes the scene and characters on which the curtain rises, they define the roles the actor is now to play. They make clear to the individual and to others that a new era, a new status in life has begun. They point always toward the future, defining and initiating the stage of life that follows. They "signify the change from one position to another in society . . . [and] modify the participant's self-concept so that the new role . . . may not be incongruent with the self."[17]

Ministry is concerned with the way we live out our lives. Through our rites and sacraments, we affirm that the way we live is as important to God as it is to us. Among the most ancient rites and sacraments of church and synagogue are those celebrated in conjunction with some of the transition events described in Chapter 4.

LIFE EVENT	SACRAMENT OR RITE
Birth	Infant Baptism/Circumcision/ Dedication of Infants
Puberty	Confirmation/Bar or Bas Mitzvah/ Believer Baptism
End of Schooling	Ordination/Licensure/Baccalaureate
Household/Marriage	Matrimony/Religious Vows
Parenthood	Baptism/Circumcision/Dedication
Empty Nest	
Retirement	
Infirmity	
Death	Funeral/Requiem Mass

"Because of our traditions," says Tevye, "everyone knows who he is and what God expects him to do."[18] The purpose of these rites of passage is in part *anamnesis*, literally *not forgetting*. More is at stake than merely remembering. In each of life's transitions we are dealing with matters of such importance that we are in peril if we forget their significance, if we forget who we are and what God expects us to do.

For some of life's transition events, traditional rituals serve as religious rites of passage. They mark out clearly who we are and what God expects of us. They inform others of our new status in life and spell out how they are to behave toward us. For other transition events, especially those associated with later life, there is little in the way of ritual that can serve as a religious rite of passage.

Infant baptism, circumcision, and other rites for the dedication of children are usually observed within days after birth. They mark the beginning of life and call attention to the child's dependence upon others for sustenance, protection and nurture in the faith. They invoke God's providence for the new human and for the parents charged with the child's care and upbringing. Often they make provision for the child's well-being, should the parents be unable to carry out their charge, by designating godparents or assigning responsibility to the congregation. These rites look forward; they anticipate the time when the child will claim and affirm the parent's faith.

Confirmation, bar or bas mitzvah, and believer baptism traditionally celebrate the transition from child to adult. These rites mark the beginning of a new era of life and redefine the individual's status. Claiming the parent's faith as one's own, the individual, usually an adolescent, now stands beside others as an adult member of the faith community. These rites also look toward the future. They affirm adult membership in the congregation, but acknowledge the need to grow into the fullness of faith, and so invoke God's watchful help for the journey that lies still ahead.

The ordination of those entering ministry or priesthood can be considered a paradigm of transition rites for the completion of formal schooling. The origins of licensure and certification for other crafts and professions probably lie in older rites for the ordination of priests and the licensing of physicians and lawyers. Baccalaureate belongs more to school than to church, and is today little more than a religious blessing on a secular occasion. Nonetheless, it calls attention to the religious dimensions of the transition from schooling to work as one's principal occupation. As with other rites of passage, ordination, licensing, and baccalaureate focus on the future. Through word and action, they recognize the individual's new status and call upon God to bless the pursuit of a new vocation.

Holy matrimony marks the passage of two individuals into a new life together and declares publicly their obligation to be faithful to each other and to establish a household together. The vows taken by those entering religious vocations are for them the counterpart to marriage vows. Promising celibacy, they choose "marriage to Christ" rather than fidelity to a marriage partner. Vowing poverty, they choose not to establish a household, not to own worldly goods. The rites for both marriage and religious vocation look forward. The worshipers invoke God's blessings and nurture and offer prayers for the individuals' faithful life in their new estate.

Infant baptism, circumcision, and other dedication rites usually call attention to the function of parents in the nurture and religious development of the young. Participation with our children in these rites therefore marks our passage into parenthood. In welcoming the child into the faith community, these rituals define the future for parents as well as child. They proclaim the parents' new status and invoke God's aid in carrying out their new responsibilities.

Rites that mark children's passage from schooling into work, and from single life into marriage, similarly mark their parents' passage into the "empty nest" era of life. These rites celebrate the child's transition to adulthood, but provide little guidance for the parents' concurrent transition. The participation of grandchildren in the rites associated with birth similarly marks our passage into grandparenthood. Traditional rites usually do not formally include the grandparents as participants, however. By this omission, they neither mark the concurrent transition in the grandparents' lives, nor address the grandparents' role in the child's nurture.

Historically, rituals developed over long periods of time as social expectations and religious meanings gradually took form around major life events. Because rites of passage always look forward to a new status, the absence of religious rituals at the major transitions of later life tends to reaffirm our fears that there is nothing left to look forward to. In the absence of a suitable rite of passage, the meaning and purpose of our lives is dependent upon a popular attitude that denigrates old age. The absence of religious or social norms for the later years leaves us uncertain about the roles we are to play in the acts to come. As a result, we are left to improvise throughout maturity and infirmity until the final transition of death. In the absence of clear directions we may lose our way and wander aimlessly.

In a half century or less, the empty nest has come to be a significant transitional event in millions of lives. A rite of passage for this transition is sorely needed. Like other such rites it must look toward the future rather than the past. It must mark our movement into a new era or epoch of life, and must establish norms for our behavior. It must tell others who we are, now that the children are grown, and what to expect of us.

Admitting that it runs against the grain of a technological society, Eugene Bianchi proposes that those who have reached this threshold "make their lives more contemplative within the context of active, worldly endeavors."[19] To be sure, the awareness of time's passing that often dawns on us in the middle years, does sometimes send us searching for our roots, for values other than those of the marketplace, for some sense of life's purpose. If, in life's afternoon, we are called to the transformation of our society, then a transition rite for the empty nest ought to call us to such searching.

In the past, women who had completed child rearing often increased their activities as volunteers in church and community efforts to help those in need. Today, many women resume careers or continue their education once the children are in school all day. Others follow their example once the nest is empty. Both men and women, once careers are going well and children's needs have grown fewer, yearn for a new challenge. A rite of passage for this time in life ought to call us to turn our attention toward making this world a fitter place for all. It ought to urge us to put education or career to the service of a more complete human fulfillment.

By the time we have reached the empty nest, we have devoted years to rearing children. A rite of passage for this time in our lives ought to call us to employ our skills of nurture and caregiving for the benefit of the wider community. Here we might be instructed by the practice in some churches of setting apart deacons, like those chosen by the early church (Acts 6:1-6), for ministries of service and compassion. In many traditions, the setting apart of members for the office of deacon symbolizes a turning of life from self toward others.

Rites are powerful in their ability to affirm the value and purpose of human life. The absence of a religious rite tends to label a life transition as lacking in religious significance and consequence. This is particularly the case in the absence of a religious ritual for retirement. Business rituals, such as the presentation of a gold watch, have generally disappeared as the number of people retiring annually has increased rapidly. The absence of a religious rite tends to affirm society's judgment that the event is so common or of such little consequence as to be not worth marking.

The ordination of lay elders, as practiced by many Reformed churches, could be the paradigm for a rite of passage into maturity. In the past, lay elders were usually older men. Many were retired and had more time to devote to church governance, particularly to regional and national church bodies. Today, the elders of a congregation usually include women and men of widely varied ages. Nonetheless, the office recognizes that "there were in Old Testament times elders for the government of the people,"[20] who helped govern (Numbers 11:1-30), rendered judgments and executed justice (Deuteronomy 21:18-21), and witnessed contracts (Ruth 4:1-12).

In ancient times, the city's elders could usually be found near the city gates. Adults and children came to learn from them the ways of life and traditions of the people. Women and men sought their judgment in settling disputes. They were not formally chosen for this function, however. The community accepted their leadership and influence partly because of tradition and partly because of their experience, skill and wisdom. Mature adults continue to play similar roles in many organizations and communities. That others do not play such roles does not indicate a lack of competence or readiness to do so. Rather, it reflects a lack of clarity, on their part and by society, about the roles they are to play at this stage of life.

Holy unction, ritual anointing, is primarily a sacrament of healing, entrusting the individual to the greater healing which can come only from God. It is best known to Protestants as a rite associated with one's final illness and approaching death. Administered together with the sacraments of final penance and final communion (*viaticum*), when death is imminent, it is part of the "last rites" in preparation for death. "In such cases, the anointing is for the world to come, an anointing to the glory of life after death."[21]

A ritual derived from holy unction might serve to mark the individual's transition from the relatively active years of maturity to the more dependent years of infirmity characterized by frailty or final illness. It should, like other rites of passage, celebrate the closing of one life stage and the beginning of another. It should proclaim to others the individual's new status and remind the older person of the norms for behavior in this new state.

The rite for infant baptism affirms the child's role as care receiver, as it does the parent's role as care giver. Because the coming years will be characterized by dependence upon others for support and care and for life's essentials, a rite for entrance upon infirmity should affirm the receiving, as well as the giving, of care within the bosom of the religious community. Because the final illness is the last stage before death, such a ritual should also focus upon death as an event to be welcomed rather than feared (Romans 8:38-39, I Corinthians 15:51-57, Philippians 1:21-23). It should make clear how a Christian approaches death and how others aid that preparation.

Finally, the funeral or requiem mass marks the individual's passage from life into death. These rites witness to the resurrection, and look toward the future as they entrust the individual finally to God's everlasting love. The custom of a wake, in which family and close friends sit with the body the night before the funeral, can reinforce our awareness that one of our number is passing into a new epoch.

In reducing the funeral to something for the living rather than for the dead, however, we lose sight of its importance as a rite of passage, conveying the individual into a new status in the faith community. Like other rites of passage, the funeral should retain its function of identifying the roles the individual is now to play, and declaring the norms for this era of our common life.

Worship is the church's central activity, "the center from which all other actions of the church take their meaning."[22] Through rite and sacrament, we experience God's love in word and action, and offer our lives to God in faithful response. Liturgies differ among various communions, but in one form or another, the church's traditional rituals celebrate the major transitions through which life moves. As life has lengthened, the transitions of the later years have become more common. As we understand better the nature of those transitions, our liturgies will reflect a better understanding of God's intentions for maturity and old age.

Ministry can function in the life of the church much as does artistic direction in the life of the theater. We can look for the potential in every life play, every individual performance. We can seek in each act, each scene, that which is essential to the whole. We can devote as much skill and care to the performance of the later acts as we do the earlier ones. We can nurture the varied ways individuals play their roles within each act. We can encourage each person to realize the possibilities in every scene change, every entrance and exit. We can urge each actor to reach for the highest fulfillment of his or her God-given potential.

NOTES

1. OLDER AMERICANS ACT OF 1965, AS AMENDED (Washington, DC: U.S. Department of Health, Education, and Welfare, Administration on Aging, July 1979), 2-3.

2. Abraham H. Maslow, MOTIVATION AND PERSONALITY (Second Edition) (New York: Harper and Row, 1970), 35-51.

3. *Ibid.*, 149-180.

4. Thomas Bradley Robb, THE BONUS YEARS (Valley Forge: Judson, 1968), 77.

5. Dorothy Soelle, THE STRENGTH OF THE WEAK: TOWARD A CHRISTIAN FEMINIST IDENTITY (Philadelphia: Westminster, 1984), 28-29.

6. Erik H. Erikson, CHILDHOOD AND SOCIETY (Second Edition) (New York: W.W. Norton, 1963), 268-269.

7. Erik H. Erikson, INSIGHT AND RESPONSIBILITY (New York, W.W. Norton, 1964), 132-134.

8. C. J. Jung, MODERN MAN IN SEARCH OF A SOUL (Translated by W.S. Dell and Cary F. Baynes) (New York: Harcourt, Brace & World Harvest Book, n.d.), 109-110.

9. Paul Tournier, LEARN TO GROW OLD (New York: Harper & Row, 1972), 11.

10. Eugene C. Bianchi, AGING AS A SPIRITUAL JOURNEY (New York: Crossroad Publishing, 1982), 2.

11. H. Richard Niebuhr, CHRIST AND CULTURE (New York: Harper Torchbooks, 1956), 233.

12. *Ibid.*, 190-229.

13. See James J. Callahan, Jr., "Case Management for the Elderly: A Panacea?" in JOURNAL OF AGING AND SOCIAL POLICY, Volume 1, Numbers 1/2, (Binghamton, NY: Haworth Press, 1989) 181-195; also R. Steinberg and G.W. Carter, CASE MANAGEMENT FOR THE ELDERLY (Lexington, MA: Lexington Books, 1983), and B. Davies and D. Challis, MANAGING RESOURCES TO NEEDS IN COMMUNITY CARE (Brookfield, VT: Gower, 1986).

14. Draft Standards for Case Management (Washington, DC: National Institute on Community-based Long-term Care, National Council on the Aging, December 1987), 1.

15. Evelyn Underhill, WORSHIP (New York: Harper Torchbooks, 1957), 32-33.

16. W. Lloyd Warner, THE FAMILY OF GOD: A SYMBOLIC STUDY OF CHRISTIAN LIFE IN AMERICA (New Haven: Yale University Press, 1961), 343.

17. Theodore R. Sarbin, "Role Enactment" in ROLE THEORY: CONCEPTS AND RESEARCH by Bruce J. Biddle and Edwin J. Thomas (New York: John Wiley and Sons, 1966), 198.

18. FIDDLER ON THE ROOF, Book by Joseph Stein, Music by Jerry Bock, Lyrics by Sheldon Harnick (New York: Crown Publishers, 1964), 1.

19. Eugene C. Bianchi, AGING AS A SPIRITUAL JOURNEY (New York: Crossroad Publishing, 1982), 2.

20. CONSTITUTION OF THE PRESBYTERIAN CHURCH (U.S.A.), PART II, BOOK OF ORDER (1983-85 Edition) (Office of the General Assembly, 341 Ponce de Leon Avenue NE, Atlanta, GA 30365), 32 [G-6.0301].

21. THE BOOK OF CATHOLIC WORSHIP (Washington, DC: The Liturgical Conference, 1966), 758.

22. Donald MacLeod, PRESBYTERIAN WORSHIP: ITS MEANING AND METHOD (Richmond: John Knox, 1965), 18.

Index